# DEVILS IN OUR FOOD

## Christine Thompson-Wells

BA, Dip of Teaching, MACEA
(Majors in Psychology)
Professional Educator, Author & Independent Writer

We support Diabetes Type One & Motor Neuron Disease. 10% of the net sales will be divided equally between both charities.

# Books for adults:

Making Cash Flow
39 Days & 39 Steps to Debt Recovery
How to Reduce Stress
Beat Stress in 20 Seconds
Stop Family Violence Now
Discover Your Selling Power
Selling Made Easy
How to Find Your Mind of Gold – Mind Power
The Game of Money & How to Play It
The Golden Book of Whispering Poems
How to Create Easy Flower Arrangements
How to Create Easy Wedding Bouquets
Healing & Wellbeing from Flowers & Plants

*More adult books are written and will be released in the future*

# Audio books

Whispering Australian Native Flowers
Whispering Wildflowers
Whispering Roses
Whispering Lilies
Whispering Orchids
Devils In Our Food

# Children's books

Will Jones Space Adventures & The Money Formula
Will Jones Space Adventures & The Money Formula –
The Play
Will Jones Space Adventures & the Zadrilian Queen
Will Jones Space Adventures & The Children
of the Black Sun
Seven more books in the Will Jones Series
will be released.

*I have no financial or vested interested in any food company or food outlet. This book has been written through the collection of observational research and with a concern for the wellbeing of all people who do not have the time to collect this valuable food information.*

*Food manufacturing companies need to be brought to account for the ingredients and additives they put into their manufactured food products. We now know many additives are making people ill and will become sick in the future. There will be more pain and heartbreak, higher medical bills and more fatalities.*

## Disclaimer

This is not a medical book and should not be used as such. The contents have been developed through observational theory and research (observational psychology). Information is also drawn from scientific literature, web search and personal enquiry. While all care is taken, the information is not warranted as accurate. Additive numbers, E Numbers and ISN numbers are continually changing and being updated. At the time of writing this book, the Additive Numbers were current.

The diagrams are for information and to enhance the meaning of the written text.

Statements, information and ideas within this book are for education purposes only. The text presented allows the reader to draw their own conclusions on the content offered.

Always consult with your doctor for possible illness or underlying illness.

Before dietary investigation, consult a dietician with an interest in food intolerance or food related diseases and disorders.

Christine Thompson-Wells (MSI) Australia and Books For Reading On Line.Com, cannot be held liable for any errors or omissions.

*I have no financial or vested interested in any food company or food outlet. This book has been written through the collection of observational research and with a concern for the wellbeing of all people who do not have the time to collect this valuable food information.*

*Food manufacturing companies need to be brought to account for the ingredients and additives they put into their manufactured food products. We now know many additives are making people ill and will become sick in the future. There will be more pain and heartbreak, higher medical bills and more fatalities.*

## Disclaimer

*Hypothesis for writing this book ~
People can make intelligent decisions
about the food they eat once they
understand how the manufactured
chemistry of the product affects their
health.*

*Respect for our food has been lost.*
*It's now time to have that respect back into our life force.*
*For all people, respect for food is paramount for individual good health and wellbeing.*
*Food manufacturers have been dictating to the consumer, through bright and gimmicky advertising, to sell their products through visual appeal that does not always represent the quality and goodness of the product portrayed on its packaging image.*
*From the manufacturers, it's now time for honesty of the product and in the ingredients in the food we eat.*

*Prior to 2002, corporate food manufacturers could add up to 10 percent of food additives into their products.*

*From 2002, food manufacturers were allowed to put 5 percent of food additive into their products.*

*A food manufacturer does not have to declare food additives on the food information panel of the product if the additive is below 5 percent.*

*If the additive is 4.99 percent you will not know if the food you are buying or eating has a food additive or multiple additives!*

Copyright© 2019 MSI Australia
All rights reserved.

ISBN: 978-0-6481884-5-2

Published by Books For Reading On Line.com
Under license from MSI Ltd, Australia
Company Registration No: 642923859
NSW, Australia
See our website: www.how2books.com.au
Or contact by email: admin@booksforreadingonline.com
Covers and Copyright owned by MSI, Australia

MSI acknowledges the author and images used in this book.

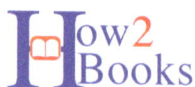

How2
Books

# The Devil's Additives

Synthetic additives are manmade substances put into our food

Made of petrol and oil of crude

These mighty **devils** are not helpful at all

They only go to make our bodies and brains fall...

And it's all because the demands are high

For food manufacturers to create sales that reach the sky!

No accountability they take – it's just big profits they make...!

They call this stuff they sell food, but it's not food at all, it's really just fake...

More **devils** will be added as technology advances

With the humble customer unaware as they buy what they need while in 'additive name' trances...

With words so long they cannot be said, they were only meant to be heard by the dead

Liver problems, gout are just some to mention, without birth defects and hypertension

It's now time to stop this abuse and to give to the customer real food for the money they pay

Without the substances having too long a name and too difficult to say...

# Content                                    Page

## Chapter One – Sugar                        1
*The devil of sugar*

- ❖ Why is sugar a devil, a toxin and poison?
- ❖ The journey of the sugar crystal
- ❖ Leg ulcers
- ❖ Young offenders
- ❖ Brain hunger
- ❖ Vitamin B
- ❖ Other possible associated negative thinking
- ❖ outcomes from eating sugar
- ❖ Symbiotic bacteria – your microbiome
- ❖ Food chemistry
- ❖ Carbohydrates
- ❖ Complex carbohydrates
- ❖ What is a complex carbohydrate?
- ❖ What is an empty carbohydrate?
- ❖ Lipids
- ❖ Proteins
- ❖ Parents can create addiction in their child or children
- ❖ The young brain of a baby or child needs Protection Tom's story
- ❖ Here's what happens
- ❖ Dopamine is released once the by-product of a sugary food is eaten or drink is swallowed
- ❖ The start of the attack
- ❖ Sugar, the opiate
- ❖ Toxins build-up in the human system
- ❖ What is stress?
- ❖ Now, the build-up of dopamine
- ❖ More dopamine is released
- ❖ The intake of poisons and toxins start to create bad eating habits
- ❖ Dopamine and adrenaline
- ❖ Extra pressure is felt by the child as more hormones are released
- ❖ The brain can go into starvation – the legacy of junk food
- ❖ Devils to look for in children's drinks and food
- ❖ The children
- ❖ The devil
- ❖ The brain again
- ❖ The human gut
- ❖ The second brain

* The human brain
* The human brain including the cerebellum
* Continuing with the second brain idea
* The gut/brain connection
* Sweeteners
* Mouthfeel
* Your memory
* Your brain's 'pleasure centre'
* Opiates
* It's not over yet, then the devil works on:
* Sugar is an opiate
* Love
* Marketing and income
* The 'Bliss Point'
* The 'Bliss Point' sugar
* The devil's persuasion
* Your notes

## Chapter Two – *Trans*-Fats                 58
*The devil of trans-fats*

* Saturated fats – low density-lipoprotein or (LDL)
* Unsaturated fats – high density lipoprotein or (HDL)
* *Trans*-fats
* The devil in *trans*-fats
* Hydrogenation and *trans*-fat
* Palm oil
* Other names given to palm oil
* Coconut oil hidden devil or not – the experiment
* Further research on coconut oil
* *Trans*-fats – the development of the devil
* Molecules and how they work
* Saturated fat
* Unsaturated fat
* Polyunsaturated fat include
* Omega 3 foods include:
* Omega 6 foods include:
* *Trans*-fat – the unhealthy, saturated fat
* Fats identified
* Unsaturated fat and *trans*-fat
* *Cis* hydrogen atoms
* *Cis* hydrogen atom cells – double bond
* *Trans-fat*
* Effects of eating too much *trans*-fat
* *Cis* vs *Trans*
* A chemistry approach

❖ *Trans*-fat
❖ *Trans*-fat and your body
❖ Further brain research
❖ *Trans*-fat and glia
❖ The human brain
❖ Your bodily system and *trans*-fat Molecule of unsaturated fat A healthy adult human brain showing the molecule of unsaturated fat and healthy neuron connections
❖ *Trans*-fat and neuron connections
❖ *Trans*-fat again
❖ The human brain suffers
❖ The human brain under strain
❖ Children's brains and *trans*-fat
❖ Following on with the scenario of the child's brain from page 22
❖ *Trans*-fats
❖ Food additives are now added to the treat
❖ Devils come in different colours and food packaging
❖ The brain of a child when it's been eating and drinking at a fast take away food outlet – the scenario, the reality an overloaded child's system
❖ Additives do their deed
❖ Giving you some idea of how additives work
❖ Additives
❖ Starting with additive numbers in the diagram on page 108
❖ The young offenders
❖ The devils gather
❖ Through life – a young person's reaction to *trans*-fat – as the child matures, habits are established – the scenario becomes a way of life
❖ Age + *trans*-fat = poor health and ageing
❖ Your physical inside body is older than your years
❖ A healthy blood flow
❖ Healthy blood circulating around and through your body
❖ The devil in the *trans*-fat
❖ *Trans*-fat is not body friendly – it is the devil
❖ Your brain and the brains of our future generations
❖ Our planet
❖ No requirement on *trans*-fat labelling in Australia
❖ Margarine – possibly the biggest *trans*-fat devil
❖ Doughnuts – a devil and a killer
❖ Moving forward
❖ Australia
❖ Foods with *trans*-fat as an ingredient or foods cooked in *trans*-fat
❖ Children eating *trans*-fat – the unseen devil
❖ A child with a healthy brain loves to learn, play and have fun

- ❖ The accumulation of sugar, trans-fat as a child eats a takeaway meal
- ❖ The 'bliss point'
- ❖ The 'bliss point' – fats
- ❖ Visual impact
- ❖ The visual sensations as you imagine eating food
- ❖ The 'Bliss Point' reaching its goal
- ❖ Marketing enhancing the 'bliss point'
- ❖ Devils have negative side effects
- ❖ Your notes

## Chapter Three – Table Salt, Caffeine and Rice 134
*The Devils of table salt, caffeine and rice*

- ❖ Salt
- ❖ Fast running table salt
- ❖ Table salt is a devil
- ❖ Natural caffeine
- ❖ 9 Side effects of too much caffeine
- ❖ Synthetic caffeine – a devil
- ❖ The flying bottle
- ❖ Additives devils in soft and children's drinks
- ❖ Rice and arsenic
- ❖ The 'Bliss Point' salt, caffeine and rice
- ❖ Table salt
- ❖ Caffeine and synthetic caffeine
- ❖ Rice
- ❖ The 'Bliss Point'
- ❖ The devil's persuasion
- ❖ Your notes

## Chapter Four – Additives 154
*The Devils of food additives*

- ❖ Understanding additive E Numbers – Europe
- ❖ Understanding additive numbers – New Zealand and Australia
- ❖ Types of food additives
- ❖ Name to become familiar with
- ❖ Controversial additives
- ❖ Collecting research
- ❖ Additives
- ❖ Devils: Colours (100 range)
- ❖ My story of 252 Potassium Nitrate and 319 tert-Butylhdroquinone (TBHQ)

❖ Devils: Preservatives (200 range)
❖ Devils: Antioxidants (300 range)
❖ Devils: More food acids (300 range)
❖ Devils: Mineral salts (300 range)
❖ Devils: Vegetable gums, thickeners, stabilisers, emulsifiers and glazing agents (400 range)
❖ Devils: Humectants also used as sweeteners (400 range)
❖ Devils: Emulsifiers (400 range)
❖ Devils: More mineral salts (400 range)
❖ Devils: Thickeners (400 range)
❖ Devils: More emulsifiers (400 range)
❖ Devils: Mineral salts (often used as anti-caking agents (500 range)
❖ Devils: Flavour enhancers, glutamates and glutamate boosters (600 range)
❖ Devils: Miscellaneous additives (900 range)
❖ Devils: Propellants (900 range)
❖ Devils: Artificial sweeteners (900 range)
❖ Devils: Foaming agents (900 range)
❖ Devils: Additional chemicals and starches (1000 – 1522 range)
❖ Continuing – the poisoning truth – Tom's story
❖ Additives contribute to ADHD and ADD behavioural problems
❖ Behavioural changes and problems
❖ The 'Bliss Point' of additives
❖ 'Bliss Point' with your, eyes, taste buds and memory
❖ Food additives
❖ Most food additives are poison
❖ The devil's persuasion - the devils in food additives

## Chapter Five – Our DNA

390

*The Devils of additives and out DNA –
our future generations*

❖ The devils
❖ DNA
❖ So what is DNA?
❖ Our genes
❖ Tampering with the DNA system
❖ In summary
❖ The devils of the future

**References** 398

**Further reading** 404

**Images** 407

# DEVILS IN OUR FOOD

**Behaviour**

Whilst the main objective of this book is to identify the destructive additives now being included as ingredients in the food we buy, it is also about how this, so called food, affects our behaviours. From the feeling of being on top of the world to feeling grossly ill after eating something that we thought was harmless and good to eat.

**My research**

Additive numbers, E numbers and ISN numbers are all one and the same. Globally, all additive numbers will soon be known as the International Numbering System for Food Additives (ISN).

I most definitely didn't expect to find the outcomes I have found when starting to write this book. For instance, I have suffered with Tinnitus for the last nine years. I have always put this condition down to stress. On a day out in London with some friends and after eating an Asian meal for lunch I felt really sick. Not wanting to miss out on the fun I kept going but knew I didn't feel myself.

I have lived with the condition for a long time now and simply dismissed it as part of life and something that I have to live with. I have tried many remedies and suggestions to make the condition tolerable but sometimes it screams in my head, while other times, it almost goes to nothing and is almost liveable.

It has taken over seven months, almost seven days a week, of intensive research on the food additive numbers alone to write Chapter Four and still I know there is more work to do. It was during this time of research that I discovered additives: 252 Potassium nitrate and 319 tert-Butylhydroquinone (TBHQ). 252 can leave a person feeling dizzy and unwell and (TBHQ) leaves a person with ringing in the ears or Tinnitus.

I've written more about this story on page 186.

Of course, to correlate a fun day out and the consumption of additives in an Asian meal will be extremely difficult to prove, but over time, it could be done.

We have now set up a separate email address to collect information about the detrimental outcomes and possible sickness caused when food additives are added to food and that food is eaten.

If you would like to forward any information onto us, please email: research@booksforreadingonline.com Please also state whether you would like your information used in future publications.

## Introduction

Many people get up in the morning and feel like they have not gone to bed. They may have thought they had slept a good, sound sleep but they are lethargic, unresponsive and struggle to find the enthusiasm for the day they are about to live through. Do you, or have you felt like this?

This condition may be connected to the food you are eating or have eaten. Please also think about the daily amounts of caffeine or if you are a smoker, the nicotine you are ingesting or your alcohol consumption or the food additives consumed.

The food we eat creates the petrol in our tanks; our tanks need to be kept healthy and clean this allows us to get the maximum output from seriously good input...

Almost all adults have the opportunity to make the choices to eat, drink or create the habits they want to live with. We can equally eat food; drink the drink that creates bad habits that are not conducive with our body's needs for our own health and wellbeing.

The opportunity may come when a person looks in the mirror and they see the reflection they don't want to see. At that moment, the '*penny has dropped*' and they decide to do something about how they feel and look!

It's at that 'golden moment' that change can start to happen. Making positive changes aren't always easy but positive changes can be made with strength of mind, a commitment to change and the 'will' to continue.

This book is not about blame or shame; it's about taking small steps to create vitality and wellbeing in your life.

## About the author

Experiences are great teachers, sometimes I think, why did I go through that? And then say to myself, 'is the pain worth the gain?' In most instances, though not always recognisable at first, the pain and growth done, through experiencing difficult times have rewards somewhere in the future.

And so it is with the study of human behaviour. Learning about people's behaviour takes time, patience, investigation, and research into academic papers and seeing if there is a parallel or a cross-over in thought, ideas, and research outcomes. It has been many years of studying of how we each differently behave and react to each different situation that allows me to write the books I write.

This book on the **Devils in Our Food** is no exception to any of the above. Throughout the years, what has been the exception is my work, as a professional educator, with children and young adults in many schools and colleges and my work in a reform institution with young male adults. I have also gained insight by working, for a short period of time, with mature inmates at Reading Jail in the United Kingdom.

I still work as a professional educator and teach a range of subjects from anti-bullying to self-care, entering puberty and sex education. It never ceases to amaze me how receptive young minds are to new and interesting information. If given, these young minds will easily absorb both positive and negative information.

Because the study of human behaviour is indeed the study of psychology, the world we live in has a veritable wealth of information. From the way you sleep in your bed, to the way you clean your teeth or the food you eat are all aspects of the subject: psychology.

The obesity epidemic is worldwide knowledge and much publicised about. Also, the Body Mass Index (BMI) has some GPs urging people to watch what they eat. With such publicity, there still isn't much focus on 'why?' this epidemic has taken place.

There is a focus on the 'fast food' industry and the capital gain that conglomerate organisations can make by delivering unhealthy food to the masses. What has been missed in much research is the role of education and taking newly acquired and gained knowledge back to the individual.

Also a missing link in the information appears to be the role the brain plays in allowing people to develop bad eating habits through the lack of knowledge of how, they as individual's, can make a world of difference to what they eat, the way they think, feel and their wellbeing.

Education is fundamental in all walks of life, but as most Western or affluent countries become more focused on consumerism and the 'fast lane' approach to life, the food manufacturers tailor their marketing to meet the ideas of the moment. Most of the current marketing is aimed at people who have not connected to the outcomes of eating unhealthy food or for the long-term health problems and the habits created by such behaviour or to those people who may have limited resources in education and spending power. Many people think that a 'takeaway' meal will fix their hunger pains without much effort other than ordering the meal by phone or at a drive through or on the way home from work or play.

Thankfully, there is a movement to healthier eating, but it is very small with more obesity being observed and nations struggling under the burden of the obesity bill in health costs.

It is with the above that I have decided to focus on behaviour to write and develop this book. When I go into a classroom and start to speak to students about my favourite subject, the students look at me and I'm sure they are wondering, 'why is she speaking about: psychology when we should be learning about: respect or sex education?' I then explain: *'during the time of your development within your mother's womb, you learnt to suck your thumb. At first, instinct may have made you put your thumb into your mouth but your reaction to the sucking would have given you: comfort, security, satisfaction and a lot of 'feel good' feelings that your tiny brain recorded. This information was then stored in your memory and allowed you later to retrieve and use. As time progressed, the sucking of your thumb was part of the pleasure you gave yourself as you matured and became ready for your birth.'*

It is at this point that the children start to see the connection between the thoughts they have and the actions they do.

Throughout life there are connections to the thoughts we have and the actions we do. Gaining bad eating habits are a combination of thinking and action. It seems very simple here but it is a lot more complicated than this. Having said that, do you remember what I've said at the beginning of this piece of writing: '...*is the pain worth the gain?*' If you want to know about the food you eat and to know is it going to do you good by eating it? Your knowledge base may need to improve.

Not only do we all need to understand more about food and its benefits. We need to understand how the food is grown, the combined ingredients used, the method or way of preparation and if additives are added and the extraction method of additives used. It's the extraction methods in the additives you eat that can create a lot of damage in your body, your health and wellbeing.

The food we eat needs to keep us physically healthy and mentally well. The food choices we individually make will show in our mental alertness and physical abilities.

Seeing the outcome of poor food consumption is alarming. It's soul destroying to see a student who has worked hard all of the year with their studies to *'bomb out'* at exam time because their brain and mind aren't working together. Many students, though brilliant, can feel sick at the thought of examinations. Prior to an examination, I have seen students eat fast take away meals which are full of preservatives with little to no food value. They have consumed highly sugared drinks that give no long-term sustainable energy; they go on a 'high' and literally *'bomb out'* during the examination!

To take the knowledge of food and its benefits back to basics is just part of the philosophy of this book. Collectively, we all need to change first, how we think about our food and secondly, the benefits each mouthful of 'good food' gives to our body, brain and mind.

## *Devils are lurking*

It's a contradiction in terms to put the words: devil and food together and why is this? The word devil conjures up fear, not good to be associated with, stay away from and all things that are bad. The word devil makes us feel uncomfortable, ill at ease or don't go near.

The word food on the other hand means: nourishment, good for the body, brain and mind, comfort, health, wellbeing, longevity and many other well-meaning associations.

The original word food may have come from the word: fode or fude (Middle English) from foda (Old English or from fodo (Proto Germanic).[1] Regardless of the word origin, food is meant to keep us healthy. In the last 200 years, food has done far from that.

We are now in the 21$^{st}$ Century and we are still recovering, food wise, from the Industrial Revolution that began in the 18$^{th}$ Century. The small agricultural societies became more industrialised and small communities moved into the towns and cities; this was especially so in England and parts of Great Britain. The Industrial Revolution provided work for the masses and food was needed to keep the masses working in the newly developed factories and sweat shops; these establishments later stretched into other parts of the world.

To feed the masses and to keep the price affordable so that factory workers and their families could be fed, mechanism and machinery took over the production of food.

Baked bread from many bakeries in the Victorian era were known for their limited flour input with the bulk of the bread being made out of wood fibre. As recently as 1985, the New York Times identified a commercial

---

[1] https://www.quora.com.

bakery in the USA using wood fibre in their commercially baked breads.[2] Considering our latest knowledge, some food manufacturers haven't progressed much in the choices they make about the ingredients, additive and food impurities put into the food they manufacture.

In some areas of food choice, we may have moved on, however, the 'Devils' in the foods we eat are now more cleverly labelled and the use of scientific names combined with new branding and marketing techniques all help us to become more confused than ever about what to eat and what is healthy to eat?

The devil is indeed in the deed and it's time to uncover the true meaning of the word **'food'** and what is being sold under this label!

---

[2] https://www.nytimes.com

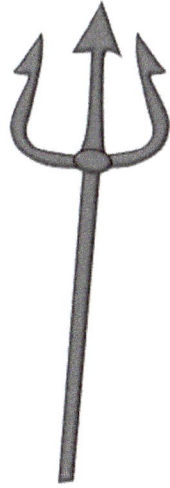

# Devils in

# Our Food

*'Unfortunately labelling of food additives is just another area where the Australian Food Regulator, Food Standards Australia, New Zealand is letting the Australian consumer down.'*

http://thefoodcoach.com.au

# Chapter One ~ Sugar

## The devil of sugar

My interest in sugar started when I was 15. One day, I said to my mother, 'I'm not eating any more sugar!' I can't say why I had made this decision or announcement, but I wanted changes in my life.' I grew up in England and the English, have had a love affair with sugar for generations, in fact, in the 19<sup>th</sup> Century it was deemed affordable, and the majority of the working class could afford it. As a teenager, my own intake of sugar became the seed that made me start to think about the real value of sugar as a food?

There are now other factors in my life that have driven me to write a book about food. In About the Author in the previous pages, I have already mentioned the obesity epidemic that hits the news daily and the numerous television programs now seen on the subject.

To begin the journey of this book, I need to retrace some of my childhood footsteps. I would be out playing with my friends and I would often see my mum walking up the street and on her way home from work; she would be carrying carrier bags of shopping packed to overflowing with groceries. I would run to help her and offer a hand however her comment would be: *'thank you, but I'm balanced and I'm nearly home...'*

Within the shopping bags there was always two pounds of sugar for use over the next week. Sugar would go on breakfast cereal, (despite the large quantity of sugar already contained within the cereal); a tablespoonful of sugar would still be added. Sugar would be added to every cup of tea or coffee, on desserts, on fruit and occasionally on a slice of bread when all other jams or spreads had run out. Sugar was sprinkled on bread and butter to reduce hiccups; I don't know if the remedy ever worked but just the same: sugar was added to the bread and butter!

I honestly don't know what made me decide to stop using sugar, but I did and from that day I have avoided processed sugar in all or most of my food.

A further awakening came into my life when our son, at the age of 10 developed Type 1 Diabetes. This is also known as Juvenile Onset Diabetes. It is not caused by a young person eating too much sugar or having too much sugar in their diet. When mentioning to someone, 'My son is a Type 1 diabetic,' the reply was: 'Oh, too much sugar in their diet or eating too much sugar...!'

Type 1 Diabetes occurs when the body's immune system, which helps to fight infections, attacks the pancreas. During the time of adjustment and retraining to work with a young diabetic, it's inevitable to learn a lot about the human system. Having to work with a strict carbohydrate-controlled diet takes a bit of getting used to but the discipline it brought into our lives has been worth the journey of awareness it has created.

From the time of my son's diagnosis until this day, my mind is constantly working and asking questions about the diets people are eating; the processed food they are consuming and the drinks they are drinking on a daily basis.

As I have previously mentioned, we are aware of the

obese situation now in many communities but logic and explanation of 'how?' and 'why?' overeating and obesity occur within an individual has not appeared to have been answered!

Before the consumption of sugar, any sweet intake made by a person would come from seasonal fruits, berries, natural honey and some grasses.

Through research, we now know that the original sugar cane was grown by the New Guinea natives at least 6,000 years BC.

The sweet liquid was sucked and chewed from the cane fibre. This rich energy-giving food, in its raw state, possesses sucrose, vitamins and minerals.

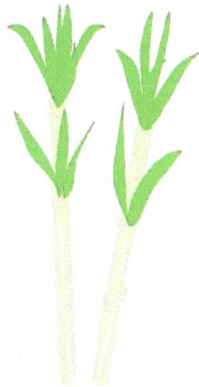

It took another thousand years for the sugarcane plant to reach other places in the world. By 5,000 BC sugarcane cultivation had spread to India, where once harvested, the sweet juice was turned into basic sugar crystals. In this form, monks and migrants could easily transport it to China, Northern Africa, and Persia. Sugar eventually reached Europe in the 11th Century.

For 400 years, sugar remained a European delicacy, spice and luxury. The fine crystals were considered to be 'white gold' and would make many sugar merchants extremely wealthy.

Christopher Columbus took sugarcane to the Americas in 1493. Sugarcane plantations were established in the West Indies and South America in the 16th and 17th Centuries. Sugar then became a vital commodity for Europe and England. In England and during the time of the Industrial Revolution and into the 19th Century, sugar intake had increased by 1,500 percent.

In the 19th Century, refined sugar was considered a necessity by the people of Great Britain, Europeans, and Americans. In the 20th Century, sugar was added to nearly every food consumed. In the 21st Century sugar is still added to cereals, breads, drinks, yogurts, health bars, juices, salad food dressings, sauces, readymade meals, frozen meals, Chinese, Indian, other Asian meals, take away meals, fast food meals and numerous other foods.

Sugar is not just a sweetener it is a poison in its refined form. Sugar also has habit forming attributes that your brain finds hard to resist.

I am not the only person who feels that it's time to make changes to what the food conglomerates and manufacturers insist on putting into the food they market to many nations around the world.

Many prominent and distinguished scientists and researchers are of a similar opinion. 'Robert Lustig of the University of California, San Francisco, famous for his viral YouTube video 'Sugar: The Bitter Truth'. A few journalists such as Gary Taubes and Mark Bittman have reached similar conclusions.'[3]

---

[3] Ferris Jabr, Credit: Nick Higgins.

It has been stated in detailed and extensive research that eating too much sugar is one of the primary causes for Diabetes Type 2, cardiovascular disease, and other metabolic disorders.

In 2014/15, six million Australians aged 18 and over were overweight. This accounts for more than a third or (36 percent) of adult Australians being obese.[4] Obesity rates among adults in the United Kingdom have almost quadrupled in the last 25 years and now around 1 in 4 falls into this category. What's more, over 60 percent of adults are classed as overweight or obese...[5] Adult obesity rates now exceed 35 percent in seven of the States in the United States of America, 30 percent in 29 states and 25 percent in 48 states. West Virginia has the highest adult rate of obesity at 38.1 percent.[6]

Given the statistics above, it's enough to put people off eating sugar, but there is more: sugar is a harmful toxin that interferes with the body's regular hormone cycles and harms organs. Referring back to my teaching, as an educator, I'm currently teaching many children in many schools in my everyday work. One of my focus areas of education is educating children as they reach puberty. From the knowledge I've gained, most educators want to develop strategies that help to protect children as they go through this stage of life. Puberty allows the body to prepare for adulthood. The time period for change in a young adult can be as long as 10 years. During this time, each individual child experiences changes; each may experience changes in different ways. Changes happen through hormones

---

[4] https://www.heartfoundation.org.au
[5] https://www.healthexpress.co.uk
[6] https://stateofobesity.org

5

kicking in to make the changes within their bodily systems.

It is now clear, through scientific investigation, sugar in its refined state, is a poison and may interfere with hormone release during the time of puberty. This interference may contribute to different and more pronounced mood swings in young adults. More investigation needs to be done, however, given the evidence so far there is a possibility that sugar, if not the culprit, it may be a contributor.

**Why is sugar a devil, a toxin and poison?**

All plants contain sugar. Sugar is needed to bring the moisture from the ground and up into the plant to keep it healthy and allow it to grow. Drawing moisture from the ground allows foliage to develop, flowers to grow and fruit to develop and ripen. This drawing up of moisture is known as photosynthesis. Photosynthesis converts light into energy; sugar allows the transition from light to draw the moisture up and through the plant. All plants work in this way.

Sugarcane has a high content of sucrose and is the main contributor to worldwide sugar production. Sugar in its natural form, as discussed previously, is not harmful to the human system; **it's the refinement of sugar that makes it toxic.**

Processed sugar is a poison and may be responsible for many of the health problems seen in the general population today. So why is this?

In 1957, Dr William Coda Martin wanted to answer the question, '*When is a food a food and when is it poison?*' His answer: '*Medically: any substance applied to the body, ingested or developed within the body which causes or may cause disease.*[7] Dr Coda Martin classified sugar as a poison *'because it has been depleted of its life forces: vitamins and minerals'.*

When sugar is processed through refinement, the leftover crystals are pure refined 'empty carbohydrates' normally seen as sugar crystals.

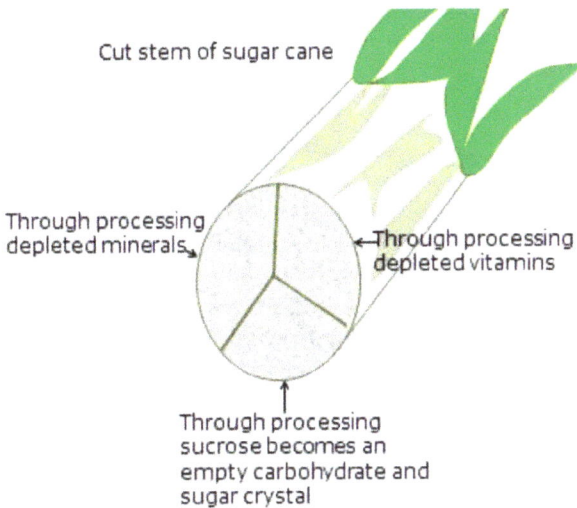

Cut stem of sugar cane

Through processing depleted minerals

Through processing depleted vitamins

Through processing sucrose becomes an empty carbohydrate and sugar crystal

The human body cannot use refined, empty carbohydrates unless the depleted minerals and vitamins are present. Accordingly, *'Nature supplies these elements in each plant in quantities sufficient to metabolize the carbohydrates in that particular plant.'*[8] It's the pure sugar eaten as 'empty' carbohydrates and eaten in above normal consumption quantities that help to contribute to the obese problems seen in today's populations.

---

[7] Dr William Coda Martin Michigan Organic News, March 1957, p. 3.
[8] Extracted Sugar Blues, © 1975 by William Dufty.

In Dr William Coda Martin's paper, he maintained: *'Refined sugar is lethal when ingested by humans because it provides only that which nutritionists describe as empty calories...'*[9] He later went on to describe how *'empty calories'* can leach from the body valuable vitamins and minerals through its demands in digestion, elimination and detoxification.

In order to satisfy the body's digestion, the intake of too much refined sugar robs the body of calcium culminating in calcium being taken from different areas of the body including the teeth and bones. Further in his paper, Dr Martin expands: *'...eating sugar in excess and eaten everyday produces over-acid; this condition will eventually affect every organ in the body.'*

**The journey of the sugar crystal**

At first, excess sugar is stored in the liver in the form of glucose (glycogen); the liver's capacity is limited. The liver, after eating excess sugar and when it becomes overloaded, will bloat. With nowhere to go, the excess glycogen is returned to the blood in the form of fatty acids.[10] Fatty acids are stored in immobile parts of the body such as the breasts, stomach, thighs, upper arms, buttocks, lower legs and ankles.

The continuous eating of sugar builds more fatty acids as the breasts, stomach, thighs, upper arms, buttocks, lower legs and ankles become larger and overloaded. Fatty acids are then distributed to active organs including the heart and kidneys. Eventually these organs start to slow down, and their tissue finally turns

---

[9] https://www.quantumbalancing.com
[10] A carboxylic acid not normally found in nature.

to fat. The whole body is affected by this deterioration and abnormal blood pressure is created.

The parasympathetic nervous system[11] with the combination of blood pressure and fatty acids in the human system, eventually affects the small brain (the cerebellum); this brain may become paralysed or inactive.

With the process of invasion of the fatty acids, the human blood circulatory, including the lymphatic system, are overrun and the quality of the red blood cells start to deteriorate thus allowing more white cells to increase. When this happens, the human body's tolerance to immunity is limited allowing for easy infection to develop. Infection may come from insect bites, virus attacks and occasional skin cuts from obscure items such as rusty nails and garden twigs and or abrasions, or intolerance to extreme heat or cold.

## Leg ulcers

I once knew a beautiful lady who has now passed. She was a biggish, English lady who was born before WWII. During the war, she and her younger brother were evacuated to South Wales in Great Britain, where they lived on a farm for the duration of the war.

This lady could cook – she could cook all sorts of delicious, sweet, English fare from: spotted dick (a type of thick dough cake made with suet, sugar and dried fruit; this is baked and served with custard. This was one of her favourites. Other delicacies were: jam roly poly, (again with sugar) and served with custard;

---

[11] While sleeping or resting, the parasympathetic system is responsible for a number of body functions including: digestion, urination, defecation, sexual arousal and reproduction.

ginger bread cake and many other 'mouth warming' delights. She worked hard for her church supplying great numbers of cakes for sale at many church functions.

Because of tradition, all cakes, sauces, and desserts had added sugar. This lady was not an exception to the rule. Large containers of sugar were always in the pantry. She may have learnt her cooking skills while living away from home during the war! Sugar gave the food 'mouthfeel'[12] and a sense of delight was experienced by the eater.

Of course, feeding people in Europe and the United Kingdom was paramount during and after WWII and people weren't interested if sugar was good or bad. The necessity for the ingredient gave the sugar producers and suppliers *carte blanche* freedom to grow more plants and process more sugar. To meet demands, sugar production became more mechanised, streamlined and sophisticated. Little marketing was needed as the product had created its own **demand** status!

In her later and final years, this lady suffered agonising pain from leg ulcers. A nurse would come to the house and change her dressings two to three times a week. The ulcers were large and continuously weeping and seeping. Regardless of the treatments given, the ulcers grew ever larger and aggressive. The lady had sleepless nights, pain and had difficulty walking; day by day, her life became ever more difficult.

---

[12] Mouthfeel is a term used in psychology which identifies the physical sensation in the mouth as distinct from the flavour of the food or drink.

'*The continuous eating of sugar builds more fatty acids as the breasts, stomach, thighs, upper arms, buttocks, lower legs and ankles become larger and overloaded with poison.*' When the human system is overloaded it reaches saturation point.

Not only is the immune system affected by an over-sugared diet but also the major functions of the brain.

## Young offenders

As an educator and having counselled and taught in many institutions, I know from observation, that students on poor diets have difficulties in learning. If I take one instance: when employed as a counsellor/educator at a young offenders' institution in the United Kingdom, the learning and lack of concentration by most of the young adults, was limited. Their main diet consisted of deeply fried potato chips, processed meats, little to no fish, with little fresh, if any, leafy green vegetables or other cooked vegetables such as carrots and cabbage.

In order for the brain to function effectively it needs to have a balance of glutamic acid[13] and other minerals and vitamins included in the daily diet. Glutamic acid is a vital ingredient found in many uncooked or unprocessed fruits and vegetables.

Fruit and vegetables, not exclusive, containing glutamic acid include:

---

[13] Both L-glutamic and glutamine acids are amino acids used by almost all living life forms and a component of protein.

| Fruit | Vegetables |
|---|---|
| • Apples | • Pumpkin |
| • Bananas | • Tomatoes |
| • Blackberries | • Artichoke |
| • Cherries | • Asparagus |
| • Grapefruit | • Broccoli |
| • Grapes | • Brussels sprouts |
| • Kiwi fruit | • Cabbage |
| • Lemons | • Carrots |
| • Limes | • Cauliflower |
| • Lychees | • Chicory |
| • Mangos | • Corn |
| • Melons | • Cucumber |
| • Oranges | • Green & red paprika |
| • Peaches | • Leeks |
| • Pears | • Mushrooms |
| • Pineapple | • Olives |
| • Plums | • Onion |
| • Raspberries | • Peas |
| • Strawberries | • Pickles |
| • Watermelon & | • Potatoes |
| • Apricots | • Radishes |
| | • Sauerkraut |
| | • Spinach & |
| | • Zucchini |

When observing the young offenders and their lack of energy it was clear that something was very wrong. The majority of the inmates were lethargic and struggled to keep attentive with most given tasks.

The environment of a prison is difficult to accept if the conviction is tough for the crime committed. This lack of understanding within the inmates also confused them. Many young people would compare their crime with that of another inmate and would consider their crime to be less when compared with others' but the sentence and conviction time was the same. The feelings of frustration and suffering from possible 'brain hunger' did not help many of the offenders.

## Brain hunger

Brain hunger or brain starvation produces lethargy, lack of concentration and a lack of commitment to any given task. Tasks were difficult for the majority of males to perform.

There had to be a common denominator that was responsible for this behaviour. As the food eaten was eaten by all inmates, without any clinical studies, it can only be my assumption that the inmates may have been suffering from, the above mentioned: *'brain hunger or starvation'.*

Having said this, as more research reveals itself, we now know that food plays a vital role in accomplished learning, not only by the inmates of a prison, but by any person attempting to grasp or learn new concepts, skills or tasks.

## Vitamin B

Mentioned on page 12 are the fruits and vegetables that contain glutamic acid and vitamin B. The brain needs to function by an orderly process. Eating the right 'brain food' allows this process to work. Eating the correct food eliminates brain hunger or brain starvation. Vitamin B also plays a key role in separating glutamic acid and the compounds which allows a controlled response[14] in the brain to happen. Vitamin B is key to good mind health, it does not add to your energy level or fuel for your body however, vitamin B plays its role by helping cells to multiply making new DNA[15] and helps the body to use the energy provided by fat, carbohydrate and the protein eaten in a regular and balanced diet.

**Symbiotic bacteria**

B vitamins are also produced by symbiotic bacteria[16] which live in the intestines. Regularly eating refined sugar (the devil) has been identified as a culprit that depletes the natural intestinal flora system which in turn, withers the friendly bacteria that eventually die, thus depleting the B vitamins produced by the symbiotic bacteria.

The consequences may lead to:

- Lethargy and a feeling of being unwell
- An inability to calculate and make specific judgement; this may be part of the cause of many road accidents!
- Premature loss of memory or the associated skills attached to the memory
- In student performance: the inability to perform at school, college or university examinations
- Industrial accidents caused through the inability to think clearly
- Short-tempered and irritable (road rage)

---

[14] The brain has centralised control over other organs or parts of the body.
[15] DNA = deoxyribonucleic acid is the molecule that carries genetic information in all human and all other living organisms.
[16] The living together by parasite and host. Anton de Bary in 1869.

- Outbursts of uncontrolled emotion and other behaviours that are uncharacteristic to the incident or event
- Erratic behaviour which are not related to any current event.

## Other possible associated negative thinking outcomes from eating sugar

- Limitations in analytical deduction and analysis
- Inability to work through simple tasks
- Lack of understanding to given instruction.

Contributing factors may include:

- The decline in health and wellbeing
- The feeling of: *'things aren't right but I don't understand why?'*
- Mood swings and mental fatigue, your brain is in starvation.

## Symbiotic bacteria – your microbiome

As a baby is born naturally through the birth canal, it picks up the microbes from its mother. After birth, it takes a further three years for the microbiome[17] to become customised and to work within the child's gut and bodily system.

Other defence structures are put into place when the baby is fed on its mother's milk and living within its environment.

---

[17] The microbiome is an ecosystem of microbes including viruses, bacteria and fungi. These live within the gut and other areas of the human body.

Eamonn Quigley, M.D., of the Houston Methodist Hospital and renowned for his research into intestinal diseases says, *'A healthy microbiome is important for health, period. The more diverse your microbiome, the healthier you are.'*

As the child grows, it eats more forms of complex food which allows more microbes to develop thus, releasing enzymes from the gut, this assists with digestion. As we grow and mature the gut microbiome becomes more complex – the friendly bacteria work with the digestive juices while extracting from the foods important vitamins and minerals.

## Food chemistry

Food chemistry consists of carbohydrates, proteins, alcohols and fats. Food chemistry is the study of the relationship of all food in both the biological and non-biological matter. Biological matter includes: milk, meat, poultry, beer and lettuce. Within biochemistry the main elements comprise: carbohydrates, lipids[18] and proteins. Not exclusive to these elements are vitamins, enzymes, minerals, flavours, food additives and food colours.

## Carbohydrates

Children are reservoirs of information. While teaching a group of eleven-year-olds the subject of carbohydrates came up. When I said to one boy, 'yes, but what carbohydrate are you talking about? Is it a complex or empty carbohydrate?' He sat in his chair and really pondered the question. Of course, the

---

[18] A lipid is a molecule that contains hydrocarbons that form the structure of living cells.

questions were answered and a debate about all types of food took place.

**Complex carbohydrates**

With complex carbohydrates the goodness of the food is left in place and little to no food processing has taken place apart from possibly a gentle and quick cook. Such foods include:

- Fresh fruit
- Fresh vegetables, lightly cooked
- Raw nuts
- Wholemeal breads
- Unprocessed cereals
- Legumes, peas and beans
- Brown rice (please see Chapter Three)

The range of complex carbohydrates, though the list seems small above is large. It would include: potatoes, sweet potatoes (yams), parsnips, carrots, onions, pumpkin, beetroot, rutabaga or (swede), beans, a large range of different fruits including bananas, oranges, apples, plums, nectarine, mango, berries of all types, pineapple, pears and more.

**What is a complex carbohydrate?**

Complex carbohydrates are contained in those foods that are fresh, with limited to no processing taking place; the un-processing of food keeps it healthy. Processing and over-processing of foods is what makes the food unhealthy and possibly poisonous.

Having said that, a complex carbohydrate is made up of lipids which contain sugar molecules, these molecules are strung together in complex chains.

Complex carbohydrates provide vitamins, minerals, and fibre. The bulk of a complex carbohydrate is made up of starches (sugars) which naturally occur as the plant grows. The naturally grown complex carbohydrate eaten in fresh and healthy foods makes the body work to break down the contained fibre, vitamins, and minerals. The work done by breaking down the food is what keeps the gut and body healthy.

## What is an empty carbohydrate?

The empty carbohydrate is a manufactured and engineered chemical sold as a food source, in this instance, sugar. Empty carbohydrates are found in refined and processed foods such as chocolate and chocolate bars, candy and candy bars, processed and manufactured French fries, processed and manufactured crinkle cut chips, crisps, breads, processed snacks and snack bars, many pre-prepared and take away fast foods, condensed and sweetened milks, many drink products, including milk and fruit-based drinks sold as healthy drinks for toddlers and babies. A definite devil is here. This website is worth a look if you are giving your child fruit-based drinks marketed directly for child consumption: *https://nakedwildandfree.com/children-naughty-fruit-shoot/*

## Lipids

Lipids include the oil naturally found within fresh food sources. Oils are found in natural animal fat, many grains including soy and corn. They're also found in milk, cheese, fresh meat and some oily fish. Lipids carry vitamins to the essential areas which allow your muscle and bodily processes to work. Lipids also carry fatty acid molecules, their derivatives which include:

phospholipids[19] and monoglycerides[20] also sterol which contains metabolites and cholesterol. As said, food is made up of carbohydrates, lipids and proteins. Fresh food including: fruit, vegetables, nuts, seeds, meat and fish have their lipid containing molecules left intact, even after some gentle cooking. These molecules are called *cis*. The molecule is as nature intended. The food we eat containing natural, living molecules, is friendly to our gut; we receive the life-giving energy it provides, and we remain healthy. When heavy processing of food takes place, in this instance sugar cane or sugar beet, the natural sugar liquid is extracted and heated to high temperatures changing the molecular living structure to an empty, dead molecule seen in the shape of the sugar crystal. When the molecular structure of a molecule is changed, the hydrogen within the original structure is moved into another position, this is called *trans*. There's more about molecules in Chapter Two.

## Proteins

In your body, proteins transport molecules from one location to another. Proteins are either bio-molecule or macro-molecule consisting of one or more long chains of amino acid[21] and some residue which plays a vital role in working with your body's neurotransmitter network. Proteins also support your DNA replication. *'Each gram of protein carries 4 calories.'*[22]

---

[19] A major element of all cell membranes.

[20] A group of glycerides which are elements of a molecule of glycerol connected to a fatty acid.

[21] Consists of nitrogen, oxygen, hydrogen, sulphur and carbon – the building blocks of proteins.

[22] University of Illinois, McKinley Health Centre.

**Parents can create addiction in their child or children**

Parents can encourage an addiction in their child or children! It's a frightening thought but it's the truth. In the supermarkets, I've seen parents read labels before they buy their children's food products never realising that the product they are about to buy is increasing their child's potential to become drug addicted. Clever branding and marketing help to keep selling food and drink to unsuspecting parents. When refined sugar is added to food products marketed to the child marketplace, without realising by the parent, a child can consume vast quantities of sugar.

**The young brain of a baby or child needs protection**

A child's brain is thought to be grown by the age of five. However, with current information and new research, there are new theories on this and it's thought now to be a little older. Having said that, the human brain, though grown, does not mature with full neuron pathways, neurotransmitters and synapse connections in place until the young person is in their mid-twenties.

Many forms of fruit drinks labelled as healthy for infants, young children and older children are **not** healthy.

I am going to make you aware now. If you have been in the habit of giving your child a fruit drink because they are demanding this drink, this child is already on the pathway to addiction. Such addiction may lead to other, more severe addictions, in their teenage years.

Many adults naively give infants and young children *'just a little taste'* of something sweet when they are eating food themselves. It may be a taste of ice cream, chocolate or refined and processed fruit juice. This could be a big mistake. Regardless of age, the healthy human memory records everything that happens in our lives. We may not be aware of those recordings but they are there sitting inside our heads and just waiting to be tapped into at a later date.

## Tom's story

I am now introducing you to a young child whom we'll call Tom. Tom is taken out by his dad for a food treat. His dad thinks it will be a good idea to have a fast food lunch. Outlined in the following pages and diagrams Tom is shown, through symbols, how sugar, *trans-fat*s and additives can accumulate in a child's system.

**Your scenario:** you decide to take your child out for a treat and think that visiting a fast food chain for a takeaway meal is a great idea. You may think, *'we can spend some quality time together!'* After the meal, your child may start to exhibit different behaviours. You may not realise the interaction and connection between the food your child eats, with the invasion of manufactured opiates,[23] and the behaviours your child shows; these are all part of a very common experience witnessed by adults across the globe. Tom's 'junk food' journey goes over many chapters.

Molecules and their deposits of sugar, *trans-fat* and additives within the human brain are impossible to see

---

[23] Is a modern expression used to describe substances, both synthetic and natural, to bind the opioid receptors in the brain.

with the naked eye. Therefore, the symbols are enlarged to give you some idea of how additives and processed food chemicals can build up within the human system.

**Here's what happens**

The synapses, shown below, are sparking as they should be.

1)

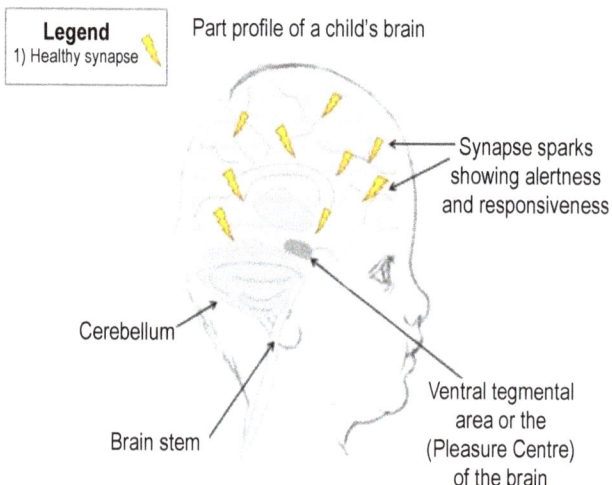

Legend
1) Healthy synapse

Part profile of a child's brain

Synapse sparks
showing alertness
and responsiveness

Cerebellum

Brain stem

Ventral tegmental
area or the
(Pleasure Centre)
of the brain

Tom, prior to being given manufactured and processed food including: ice cream, chocolate, French fries, yes, even French fries can contain sugar.

The first diagram shows Tom's healthy synapse sparks. The cerebellum, brain stem and the ventral tegmental area (sometimes referred to as the 'pleasure centre') are working together. The pleasure centre lies within the mid-brain of the human brain. (From this point on, we'll refer to the 'pleasure centre' rather than the ventral tegmental area).

The human brain is made up of many integrated parts that work together. This allows a person to live a happy life. In this diagram the synapse are healthy and sparking as they should be; this is allowing the child to learn and grow from its environment.

Synapse can be compared to the fuses in the electric fuse box that allow your home to function; it allows you to turn on a light, cook on the range, if electric or listen to the sound system. When the fuses don't work, the house doesn't function. The synapses in our brain work in a similar way. Together with synapse, the brain has neurotransmitters which work along neuron pathways.

Over the crucial years, as the brain of a child grows and develops from, conception to about five years, many parts of the brain try to adapt to the stimulus it receives. When a child is given sugary-based food it creates a hormone rush. This hormone rush allows the hormone dopamine to be released, which in turn can interfere with the working of the synapses and the neurotransmitters of the child's brain. Sugar is a stimulus, an opiate and poison.

Sugar is an inferior product that is sold to stimulate the sales of sweet, edible, unhealthy products. Research is showing more and more the damage that's being done to the human body and brain by its use.

The 'pleasure centre' of the human brain has to cope with by-products of the food or drink that has been consumed by its owner. When the 'pleasure centre' receives a stimulant, in this instance a molecule containing the sugary by-product, the pleasure kicks into gear and there is a release of dopamine from the dopamine cells within the brain's 'pleasure centre'. Dopamine is a demand hormone and the more the brain has of this hormone, the more it wants! Because dopamine is released by the intake of the by-products from sugary drinks or food, the child builds up a habit through the release of this hormone. Together with dopamine, adrenalin may also be released. The intake of sugar and the release of hormones will change the child's behaviour.

As a human species, we have not evolved to eat and drink processed, sugary foods or drinks. Sweet foods were a luxury during the time of our ancient ancestors'. They would have had seasonal sweet fruits, honey when the bees produced it or foods that were dried from a previous season. Simply, our guts do not have the enzymes to dissolve manufactured, processed, artificially sweetened food or drink that is being sold in the Twenty First Century.

**Dopamine is released once the by-product of sugary food is eaten or drink is swallowed**

While eating the fast food, the child's brain will be continually bombarded by the effects of opiates and the release of dopamine until its bodily system can take no more. The behaviour exhibited by the child will allow you to see the stress the child endures while trying to cope with artificial food and its additives.

## The start of the attack

2)

Legend
1) Healthy synapse
2) Dopamine

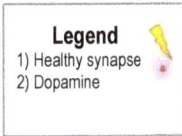

The release of dopamine as the child consumes either a sugary drink or food

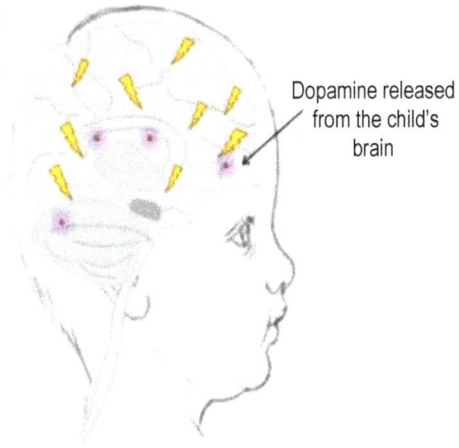

Dopamine released from the child's brain

Purple in the diagram above shows a dopamine release.

It will depend on the volume of sugar eaten and the dopamine released to the reaction and behaviour exhibited by the child. Every child is different. A child's reaction may be more severe if they have an intolerance to the product or products eaten or drinks swallowed.

Science is now suggesting, there is more than one area of pleasure within the brain and each area may react differently to the dopamine released. Differences will be exhibited in the behaviour shown by the child.

## Sugar, the opiate

The pleasure of a dopamine release in the child's brain will add to more demands from the child.

As the sugar rush hits the child's system, the demand will become greater. You may observe more drinks being wanted, extra serves of ice cream and other demands. You may see extreme behaviours as in Attention Deficit Hyperactivity Disorder (ADHD) or Attention Deficit Disorder (ADD) or other extreme behaviours not normally exhibited by the child.

Having observed children in the playground before morning tea and lunch breaks, and those with sugary-based food and drink, can show profound changes in the behaviour they exhibit. Experiencing this, I then went on to observe the type of food and drink they were consuming.

With rapid highs of sugar intake, the brain and mind are over stimulated. When the sugar rush starts to wear off, the child starts to become irritable, unhappy and possibly naughty. The child is not naughty by choice. The behaviour outcomes are the end result of a child being fed poisons, toxins and opiates. More about this on page 47.

## Toxins can build up in the human system

Every time a child is exposed to different processed and manufactured foods, their body and brain experience a form of stress. It's difficult to believe that a simple treat to a fast take away food outlet can put a child into stress, but it can. Not only is the child's body trying to cope with the toxins or poisons they have eaten, but their gut will have difficulty in processing what has been swallowed. Again, I say, 'the human body does not possess the enzymes...' required to allow empty carbohydrate/s of sugar to leave the bowel. This is not a good outcome for any child.

## What is stress?

In my research I have discovered at least six forms of stress (there's too many to go into at this point in this book). We need to have different forms of stress because **good** stress makes us get out of bed in the morning and face the challenges of the day. We don't need **bad stress** that is counter to our wellbeing and good health. Destructive additives are detrimental to both: wellbeing and good health. When the body is under attack from *devil additives*, it causes negative stress to develop. This is seen in the different and disruptive behaviours brought on by the ingesting of poison and toxins. Negative stress allows the stress hormone cortisol to be released and is usually associated with our *flight or fight* response reaction. Cortisol is produced and released from the adrenal gland. Cortisol also helps to prevent the release of substances in the body that cause inflammation.

## Now, the build-up of dopamine

The nature of dopamine is to demand. In our evolutionary past, possibly because survival was so difficult, when we experienced something good we learnt to self-gratify. We did this because it made us feel good and left us with a 'feel good' memory and experience.

# More dopamine is released

3)

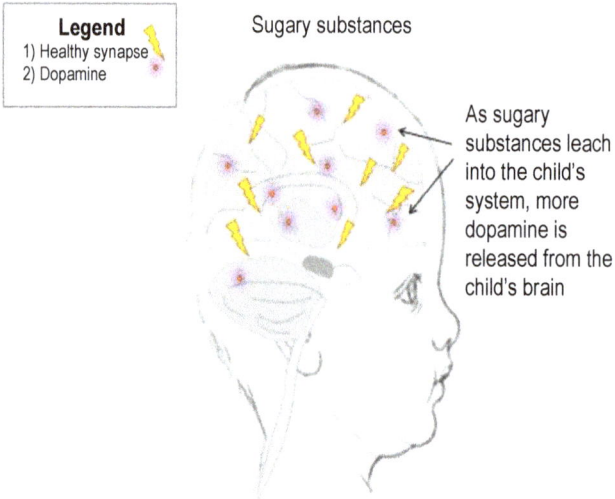

The fast food, and commercial food industries have evolved in the last fifty or so years but our body, bio-chemistry, the body's system and brain, with only minor and slight modification, are still as they were when our ancient ancestors' were living their lives.

Like today, our ancestors' would too, have released dopamine when they had experienced eating something sweet. The release of hormones would allow them to remember the sweet taste of honey, or the taste of a ripened apple, or the taste of a piece of fruit after it was plucked from the tree in the middle of the summer. They did not have disposable cash for disposable food. Can we, in the Twentieth First Century, call the manufactured substance from fast food industry and outlets or that sold in the food aisles of the supermarket, can we really call it **food?** Food is meant to replenish us and is to keep our body, brain and mind healthy. It's meant to allow us to live our lives to the full and to give us the energy we need to make the most out of every day. Most definitely, from my research to date, the majority of manufactured food does not fit into the above description. My research, please see Chapter Four, in most instances, relates to poisons and toxins in processed or manufactured foods.

**Back to our story.** A child's brain can only take so much. As parents' and carers we need to be sensitive to the reaction these poisons have on children, not only on their brains but also on their minds.

The existence of toxins may also lead the child to experience unnecessary headaches and the feeling of being very unwell.

### The intake of poisons or toxins start to create bad eating habits

Bad eating habits can start at an early age, once developed they can be very difficult to break.

Not only does a bad habit develop but the child's health will suffer through the feelings and actions of:

- Being lethargic
- Being anxious or nervous
- Being bad tempered and intolerant
- Showing a lack of concentration, therefore, learning new concepts and ideas are difficult and
- The loss of friends or the inability to make friends.

Recently released in The Telegraph, United Kingdom was an article on a boy who only ate white bread, crisps, chips and processed meat for about a decade. The seventeen-year-old, after eating this diet has now been classed as legally blind and deaf.[24] Bad eating habits need to be broken early and before the child has the mental time to establish them.

## Dopamine and adrenaline

The release of these two hormones can lead a child to appear naughty. However, because stimulated chemistry in the child's brain is taking place, the child may not be in control of the words they speak and the actions they take or do.

The child will experience the chemical changes taking place but not necessarily be aware of how? and why? they feel and act as they do!

Children are usually fed by food provided or bought by an adult.

Yes, in the majority of instances, a parent needs to take the responsibility for the food eaten and the behaviour a child exhibit.

---

[24] Dominic Lipinski/PA Lizzie Roberts, The Telegraph UK 3/9/2019

**Extra pressure is felt by the child as more hormones are released**

4)

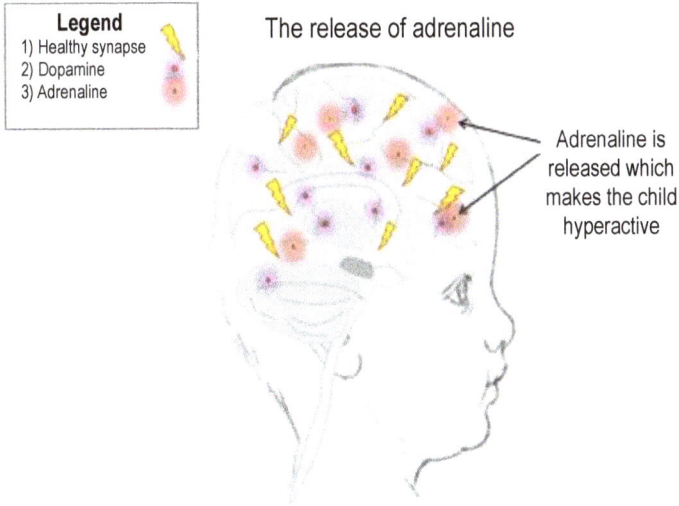

Legend
1) Healthy synapse
2) Dopamine
3) Adrenaline

The release of adrenaline

Adrenaline is released which makes the child hyperactive

Dopamine is a hormone and released from the brain. Adrenaline, like cortisol, is released from the adrenal gland that sits above the kidneys. Adrenaline is shown in pink in the above diagram. These chemicals start to flood the child's system giving it the buzz it has become familiar with.

It could now be the start of the development of a sugar and possibly a later drug habit. This type of reaction may also be the start of ADHD or ADD. All people, including children, have different tolerances to different additives and different outcomes in behaviour, health and cognitive ability. Please see Chapter Four for a full description of Food Additives.

**The brain can go into starvation – the legacy of junk food**

On page 13, I've mentioned brain starvation and brain hunger. When a child is fed on too much junk food, the child's brain can go into starvation. As a child's brain develops it needs only good, whole food. Through the lack of the value of nutritional food, a young person's brain will suffer; this could hinder a child for life which has been shown on page 30, where a child is now legally blind and deaf after eating junk food for about a decade.

An adult can make choices about the food they eat; a child must, in the first instance, be given junk, fake or manufactured food before it demands it at a future time. From the introduction of solid food, adults need to take the responsibility of creating good eating habits in their children. The other day, while out, I passed a woman who looked like a grandmother, she was talking to a very young child sitting in a stroller. The grandmother was eating an ice cream. As she spoke to the child, she scooped up an amount of ice cream with her finger and gave it to the child. The child loved the taste and waited eagerly for the next scoop. From the previous pages, you will have an idea of what the child experiences and the brain stimulation that goes on inside its head.

We all have a brain, but each brain is mechanically built differently, as one professor has said, *'No two brains are the same.'* However, many people, including children, have different tolerances and reactions to different additives, drugs and junk food. The child at a young age is not responsible for the food or drink it is given or consumes. Having said that, why expose your child to unnecessary drug taking at an early age and why subject your child, yourself and family to the outcome of naughty behaviour or the trauma after the poison is eaten or swallowed?

For future generations and at this point in our history, we do not know the long-term outcome on the human brain to the additives, over processing, poisons and toxins, including sugar, put into the foods currently sold in supermarkets, fast food outlets and food stores worldwide.

**Devils to look for in children's drinks and food – Some of the hidden devils.** Please see Chapter 4, page154, for description of food additives:

- **(202)** Potassium sorbate: **Avoid**
  Causes skin irritation, contributes to asthma and hyperactivity, ADHD and ADD.
- **(242)** Dimethyl dicarbonate: **Avoid**
  Is a dangerous toxic, synthetic yeast inhibitor used in many beverages including children's juices. Causes cancer.
- **(296)** Malic acid: **Caution** or **Avoid**
  Commercial malic acid is a synthetic derived by heating under pressure. Not recommended for children and infants.
- **(950)** Acesulfame potassium: **Avoid**
  Is a synthetic and at least 200 times sweeter than sucrose (sugar).
- **(955)** Related to aspartame: **Avoid**
- **(1401)** Acid treated starch: **Caution** or **Avoid**
  On alert in the United States and the European Union.

- **(Shellac)** Yes, the same substance that is used on furniture surfaces is also used in sweets, lollies, confectionary and other foods.
- **Corn syrup** High-fructose corn syrup (HFCS) is added to many foods that are consumed by children. These foods include: soft drinks, all forms of sweets, lollies, candy and confectionary, yogurts, salad dressings, frozen junk food, many breads, canned and small packs of preserved fruit in syrup, fruit juices, health bars that include oats and seeds. Because it takes the sweet taste to sell many products, corn syrup is cheap for food manufacturers to use so it's used as an ingredient across a great number of unhealthy food products.

Prior to the introduction of artificial sweeteners fructose was extracted from fresh fruit and vegetables. Corn syrup will increase the child's demand to want more of the sweet products its eating as the sweetness of the taste will be habit forming and could lead to obesity.

**The children**

If we are to make a different world for the children of today, who will be the adults of tomorrow, more emphasis needs to be placed on food education. It needs to be standard education that children learn about the brain, their powerful mind that works in conjunction with the brain and the acceptance that the food eaten may have both good and bad outcomes. Children are receptive and can comprehend great chunks of information. It's the adults who put on the 'learning breaks' by assumptions: *'the child is too young to learn about that...,'* or they have the assumption, *'let a child be a child...'* A child given life-skill education at an early age has a better chance of managing life as they grow older and become adults.

As the food we eat fuels the bodies we drive, why should this education ever be limited? As an educator, it has made me feel sad to have to mention such things, but it needs to said.

## The devil

Once the sugar crystal is extracted and void of its nutritional value, including the vitamins and minerals, sugar has no nutritional value at all.

Once eaten, the glucose of this empty and simple carbohydrate, without physical exercise, and as I have previously mentioned, *'... is readily stored as fat in many parts of the human body.'*

## The brain again

Many people do not understand the significance and importance of the human brain. If you look at any school national curriculum, the brain is rarely mentioned, brain storming is mentioned, but the brain appears to have such little significance and yet children are encouraged to learn at school, and some have extra curricula activities to learn and achieve most of the time. Parents even marvel at the brilliance of their five-year-old as they recite the alphabet or learn their numbers. And yet, the brain, synapses, neuron transmitters and neuron connections that allow this organ to work, have barely a consideration by educators and parents.
Like so many manmade engines that have moving or connecting parts, the human brain is similar; however,

when we start to look at the human mind in conjunction with the human brain that then takes us on another exciting journey.

The brain needs to work to allow the mind to work that's a fact, as the children in my classes often say: *'…if your brain doesn't work, you don't work, Miss.'*
The human body and brain need to work together as one finely tuned piece of human technology. Excessive sugar intake interferes with this technology.

## The human gut

The human gut and brain work in unison, if they did not, how would you know when you had a stomach upset or had a reaction to the food you had eaten? Your gut lets you know continuously if it is happy or unhappy.

Science, technology, and the human mind are great working partners. We are now discovering more information about the complicated systems of our bodies. The role the gut plays and the significant roles of your brain and mind and how they all work together.

In 1996 the hormone ghrelin was discovered. *'Ghrelin is one of the main hormones to stimulate hunger.'*[25] Ghrelin communicates between the gut and the brain letting the brain know when the body needs food. If overstimulated, extra ghrelin release may contribute to weight gain. Ghrelin is a growth hormone-releasing peptide.[26]

---

[25] Ananya Mandal MD https://www.news-medical.net
[26] Peptides are short chains of amino acids.

## The second brain

I need to point out here, you have only one brain and that sits inside your head. The brain is divided into distinctive parts: the left and right hemispheres. Between the right and left hemispheres there lies the corpus callosum. At the lower back and at the base of your skull, is the cerebellum. This also sits at the back and base of your brain. The term 'second brain' relates to your gut.

Please take some time to look at page 39 and see what exists inside your head.

a) *The left and right hemispheres:* these areas are sometimes called the new brain. These parts are a later adaption to the original brain. The hemispheres are made up of glial cells which are seen as a whitish, greyish mass and form the shape of the walnut commonly seen in many illustrations or pictures of the brain. Like all other parts of the brain, glial cells need to be kept healthy. These cells provide nutrition and protection for the neurons they protect. Neurons and neuron pathways work with synapses inside the glial and produce electronic waves. These waves help you to formulate ideas, make plans and to effectively live your life. The electricity from the waves allows you to think, make logical assumptions, work out dilemmas, come up with ideas and form the creation of your mind.

b) *The corpus callosum* contains a mass or neuron pathways that allow information to travel from your left to right hemispheres and vice versa. This is why the right side of your brain operates the left side of your body and the left side of your brain operates the right side of your body.

Inside your head, many more components sit under the glia cap. Your memory, spatial awareness, emotions and other important parts which allow you to successfully live your life are protected and working for you within your brain's environment, scaffolding and within the cap.

To keep your brain operating in this way it takes a significant amount of energy from the food you eat. In some instances, with variation, up to 65/75 percent of the food energy is used in synapse production and for relaying information.

c) *The cerebellum* also plays a pivotal role in how you move and the actions you take. The cerebellum allows you to use your gross motor skills when you want to drive your car or go for a walk. It also allows you to use your fine motor skills when you sign your name, write a letter or create a water colour or painting.

A child's brain works in a similar way, but it still is developing and maturing. The child is also on a major journey in learning. It's learning about its environment and the world in which it lives.

Like all parts of the human body, both in the adult and child, the brain will only work effectively if it is treated with respect and given the correct fuel in the food that's eaten, and the drink consumed.

# The human brain

## The left and right hemispheres of the human brain

5)                   Top view - human head

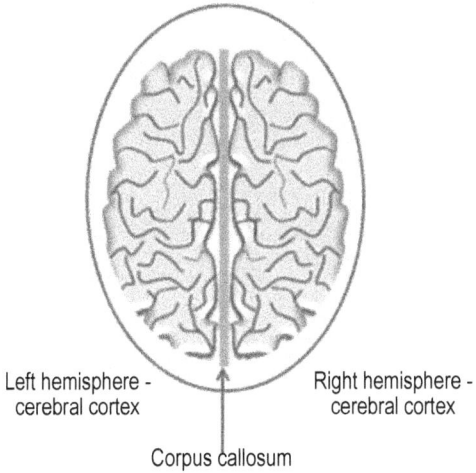

Left hemisphere -
cerebral cortex

Right hemisphere -
cerebral cortex

Corpus callosum

## The human brain including the cerebellum

6)                   Side view of the
human head and brain

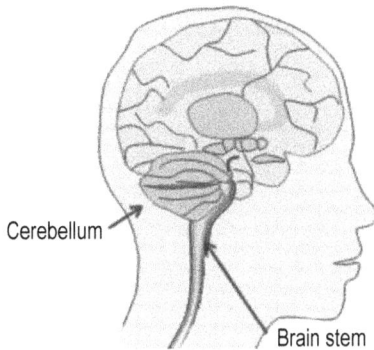

Cerebellum

Brain stem

## Continuing with the second brain idea

The second brain idea has been developed because of the communication between the gut and the brain; so how does this work? Connected are 100 million neurons that connect the throat, bowel and rectum to the brain. Each is in communication with the brain giving you constant information:

- 'I'm hungry'
- 'I'm full'
- 'I'm thirsty'
- 'I need to go to the bathroom'
- 'I have stomach cramps'
- 'I feel sick'
- 'I need junk food'
- 'I need fatty food'
- 'I just want chocolate'
- 'I want more sugar in my coffee'
- 'I need lots of salt on my chips' or
- 'I need to eat some fruit'
- 'I need to eat green food, my body is telling me this'
- 'I need to eat fish' or
- 'I need some nuts in my diet'.

Each mouthful of food eaten or drink consumed eventually the particles or residue in the form of molecules find their way into the blood stream; some of which are then transported to the human brain.

The gut is also called the 'second brain' because 'gut reactions' can affect your moods, actions, mental state or personality.

*'Studies have revealed that 70 percent of the neurons outside the brain and spinal cord are located in the gut.*

*The connection between those neurons and the central nervous system is known as the gut-brain axis, a two-way communication channel that transmits information from the brain to the intestines and vice versa.'* Rene Ebersole, independent journalist. USA.

## The gut/brain connection

7)

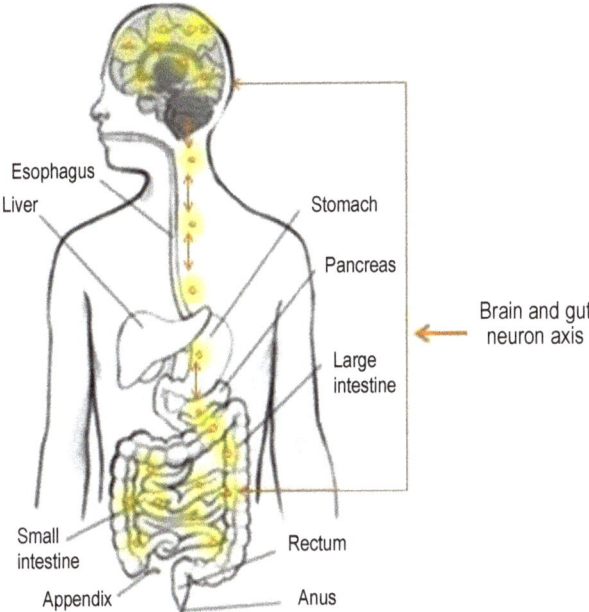

Esophagus
Liver
Stomach
Pancreas
Brain and gut neuron axis
Large intestine
Small intestine
Appendix
Rectum
Anus

Image courtesy, minus adaptations,premiermedic alhv.com

In the above diagram: when a positive, healthy connection is made through the brain/gut neuron axis and vice versa, maximum health is maintained. If the microbiome, is under constant attack from an over sugary diet; it will start to die. By slowly dying, the brain/gut axis becomes weaker and the signals sent through the neuron transmitters and receptors also

41

become weaker eventually killing the microbiome and the neuron axis connection to the brain.

The gut-brain theory is still under research but the observation of each and every person, when they feel unwell, will help to justify the reactions we seem to experience when eating the wrong food or food that is contaminated, is a toxin or is over processed.

The gut biome like other living organisms has its life cycle: it grows, multiplies, defecates and dies as a natural process of life. Trillions of microbiome work daily in your gut, each has its role to play to help keep you healthy. Below are some signs that will tell you if your gut is not healthy:

1. You suffer with bad breath
2. You may suffer with tooth decay
3. You have bouts or continuous constipation
4. You may suffer with bleeding gums – your gums may bleed during the night while you are asleep
5. You may experience bloating and gas
6. You may have heartburn, reflux or other related conditions after you've eaten
7. You cannot control your weight
8. You generally feel unwell and cannot pinpoint why?
9. You feel lethargic and have little to no energy to do the things you once did
10. You have started to lose an interest in life and the goals you have set.

All of these and more experiences can be red flags; you now start to listen to what your gut is telling you.

The second brain in your gut is about relaying information to the intellectual brain in your head. It relays information when things are wrong or very wrong with your gut and your microbiome.

In some latest research, scientists are discovering that individuals harbour over 1,000 different microbial gut species that work to keep the gut healthy.

## Sweeteners

For a full understanding of the refined crystal sweeteners put into our foods we need to understand the meaning behind the names the food industry applies to each:

1. **Sucrose**: is obtained commercially from sugarcane and sugar beet. Sucrose is a nonreducing disaccharide.[27] This means sucrose is made up of two carbons: glucose and fructose

2. **Glucose**: Every cell in your body requires the use of glucose; glucose helps your cells to regenerate and helps to maintain your health. The body doesn't need synthetic, manmade glucose, it needs the glucose it extracts from whole food in fresh fruit and vegetables

3. **Fructose**: or fruit sugar is a simple ketonic monosaccharide[28] found in many plants. When fructose and glucose carbons bond together, they produce sucrose.

Sugarcane and sugar beet in their raw form provide a valuable food source. It's the processing of sugar into the crystal form that causes the damage to the human

---

[27] Disaccharide = glucose and fructose – two simple sugars are joined by glycosidic linkage.
[28] Ketonic monosaccharides are the simplest form of sugars.

system, including the brain, teeth, bones and soft tissue of the human body.

## Mouthfeel

What is 'mouthfeel?' Mouthfeel relates to the physical sensations experienced in the mouth and is distinct from the way something tastes. Mouthfeel can be seductive, enticing and even romantic. We often see, in advertising, a model unwrap part of a bar of chocolate, break a piece from the bar with her teeth and slowly with seductive and suggestive gestures, run it across her lips before actually allowing the chocolate to go into her mouth! This is about the marketing message from the food manufacturers saying: *'Eat my chocolate and you will feel and be seductive just like me.'*

Mouthfeel is associated to the sensations relating to texture and density of the food eaten or the drink swallowed. These sensations are relayed to the brain through neurotransmitters; your brain has thousands of neurotransmitters receiving and sending messages throughout your body every moment of the day; it's a bit like an email service but this email service is working inside your body and relaying information to your brain and then transferred on to your mind for analysis. In mouthfeel, the transmitters, which connected to your senses, are on the inside of your mouth, in your cheeks, on your tongue and on your palate in the roof of your mouth.

Mouthfeel relates to your environment, life and past experiences and can be part of your genetic makeup. Mouthfeel can relate to your visual senses in the form of colour, texture, feel and taste.

When being out for the day and we take the time to look at the culinary delights available in the French Patisserie, we may start to salivate at the thought of eating a chocolate brulée or the small pistachio cream and raspberry roulade. Your eyes see the feast of delicacies and your senses are stimulated; this information is sent from your eyes through neurotransmitters and connect to the taste transmitters in your mouth and you experience a gastronomic explosion in your mind – 'if only?', you may think!

You may become weak and submit. You may think: 'Just this once!' or you may have the strength to walk away.

Remember, it's your brain working inside your head and your brain can work very effectively to weaken you if you allow it to. Many educators will label 'the brain,' 'the brain' but there is a lot more going on inside the brain than we give it credit for. The weakness for sugary food may not be completely attributed to your mental 'weakness' or 'sweet tooth!'

**Your memory**

Your memory, of past pleasurable experiences, may also play a role in the way you consume sugary delights. The fascination of taste may link to the experience gained of a flow of energy after eating or drinking anything that has sugar as part of its menu. In other words, 'classical conditioning' as with Pavlov's dogs – your memory and the chemical messengers attached to your past experiences trigger a reaction. There is an association between two stimuli, the sweet flavour of sugar and the energy boost you had after eating or drinking the sweet combination.

In Pavlov's experiments, the dogs salivated to the sound of a bell, having learned that food would follow once hearing the sound. We are very similar when it comes to sugary foods that we have become captivated by. If you can recall walking into a shop or store that specialises in fine confectionery or fine patisserie, you will recall the sweet smell of the goodies on sale. The visual appeal of the sweet products stimulates your memory together with mouthfeel interact to allow your gastronomy to kick in. This involved interaction can overtake you when you are weak and not in control of how your mind and senses are working.

Excessive sugar intake like many other addictions is just one of the psycho-stimulant's that tempt us in our everyday lives. Of course, there is more to this than what I've briefly spoken of in this last paragraph.

**Your brain's 'pleasure centre'**

Each of us has a complex brain. Through our ancestors' handing down different parts of our DNA, that brain has evolved over the last 70,000 years of maturing and nearly 50 million years of evolution. We have no idea of how the brain will be or look at the end of the next 70,000 or million years. The brain like the human body is continually evolving and re-planning itself. We can only surmise that the brain works with the human senses and will make miniscule adjustments to adjust to the environment or experiences a person has throughout their life. Though these adjustments are continually taking place, we will not be aware of the changes during our lifetime or indeed during the lifetimes of our future great grandchildren. The brain works to ensure the survival of the species, the species being us – the human race as we are at this time.

The 'pleasure centre' area of the brain is tucked away inside the technology and architecture of the human brain. It astounds me that this 'pleasure centre', with the obesity crisis in the Western and affluent world, why this is continually missed in television programs, documentaries, and the print media! The 'pleasure centre' can be a friend or villain and knowing how to work with this brain technology can work to change people's lives for the better.

Succumbing to the demands of the brain's 'pleasure centre' is like taking the candy from a two-year-old child – this is when the tantrums begin!

If you feel you have an addiction with sugar, the journey of an addiction may have started when you were just a small child. Such a habit is going to be difficult to change unless you are prepared to put in the work to be in charge of the thoughts you have and the actions you take and the changes you want to make.

## Opiates

Like so many devils they come in many disguises. Sugar, as discussed is too an opiate (is an addictive substance that has no food value at all) it's invasive to your:

- Bodily system
- The soft organs such as
    - Liver, heart, kidneys, gastrointestinal tract and
    - Invasive to your gut and your microbiome

Sugar destroys your microbes, first they wither and then die. Once the microbes are dead, your gut's defence system is reduced, in some instances, to nothing. You may experience many forms of intestinal pain and discomfort because your defences are down. Other aches and pains will come into your joints and muscles. You may find it difficult to walk, get out of a chair, drive your car, mow the lawn and even make love when you feel the urge. Not a good price to pay for an addiction that can be instantly stopped.

**It's not over yet, then the devil works on:**

- Your brain
- Your mind
- Your physical wellbeing and
- Your future

On page 41, I've spoken and described many aspects of the gut/brain axis. Not only does your decaying microbiome affect the way your brain works but it also affects that amazingly powerful mind you have inside your head. When the microbiome is sick, so is your mind. Neither your brain or mind will work effectively until you reduce your sugar intake and sort out the good from the bad food you eat.

**Sugar is an opiate**

So, what is an opiate? An opiate is a narcotic and works on the opiate receptors to produce morphine. Opiate receptors are distributed widely in the brain, in the spinal cord and on peripheral neurons. Morphine, traditionally masks pain. However, the intake of sugar works to stimulate the release of dopamine. Dopamine is a demand pleasure hormone and traditionally used in *'fight' or 'flight'* awareness for personal survival. Having said this, dopamine works throughout the body as a chemical messenger. It works in our bodies so that other organs such as the kidneys and the natural and timely urine release can function effectively. Too much sugar in a child's or adult's diet can interfere with their natural bodily functions. It interferes with the bowel and urinating functions reducing or stimulating these functions at inappropriate times. Sugar disturbs the natural chemical balance that helps to keep the body and brain healthy.

If a person has had a life-long association with sugar – they have eaten or been given sugary drinks and food in the form of bought fruit juices, biscuits and some manufactured and previously prepared baby foods, then the possibility of knowing if they are in fact feeding themselves an opiate on a daily basis will come as a surprise.

## Love

Too much sugar can interfere with your libido and make you sluggish. You are unable to get out of bed and you lack the ability to concentrate on the jobs that need to be done. In general, your energy levels are low; you lack enthusiasm and your ability to generate new ideas does not come easily.

## Marketing and income

The global sugar trade has a worldwide value of $50 billion a year. That's worth a lot of protection to the countries who grow, manufacture or produce pre-made foods, baby foods, drinks and confectionery that require sugar as part of their ingredients. In 2017, Mars in the USA had the highest sales of 18 billion US dollars with other conglomerates showing sales in the billions.

The marketing for sweet products is fierce, deliberate and packed with seductive images. Depending on the target market at the time for the advertising; the images usually incorporate young, healthy, active people. Occasionally an older, rotund person will be employed, this being the Santa at Christmas time as seen in the traditional Mars advertisements.

Shimmering neon lights, bright billboards and colourful wrapping all present the 'must have,' and 'alive' image. The advertising colours are designed to stimulate the triggers in our brains that associate with the feelings of pleasure when eating, drinking or buying sugary products.

It has been said, that, *sugar develops a culture of materialism.'* There would seem to be a parallel to this statement. To date and from WWII, there has been a surge in consumerism.

## Teens and the sugar epidemic

*'Teenagers eat three times the safe level of sugar.'*[29]

In a paper published by Lancet, (20th July, 2019) Professor Marco Peres, based at the Menzies Health Institute, Queensland and Griffith University, said, *'tooth decay is one of the most common diseases in the world*.' He continued, '*If we are talking about dental care, we need to talk about sugar*.' Further discussed in the paper from Associate Professor Mathew Hopcraft, chief executive of the Australian Dental Association, Victoria Branch, '*...tooth decay rates in Australia reflected global numbers*.' Professor Peres continued,

---

[29] Rachel Clun, Sydney Morning Herald, 20th July 2019.

'*…we wouldn't have tooth decay without sugar, and soft drinks are the major source in the global diet.*'

## Our planet – sugary foods and drinks – their wrapping and containers

We only now look at our oceans to see the discarded food wrappers, plastic straws, bottles, tins and cartons from take away foods and drinks. Most of which would have been bought as sugary food and beverages. The demand for sugary foods and drinks to date, have given nothing back to the consumer apart from illness, disease and a large medical bill that will cripple many nations in the years to come. On the other hand, the food conglomerates continue to grow wealthy with income and profit margins beyond what most of us can comprehend.

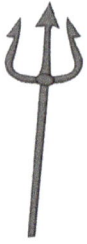

# The Bliss Point

## The 'Bliss Point' sugar

The 'bliss point' is a measured response to the food eaten. There are specific, scientific instruments that manufacture's or food conglomerates have that will allow them to measure how much sugar, fat and salt to add to a product that ensures it will sell. Also taken into the equation are the demographics, age, disposable income, (which include the socioeconomic ability of the population) and other factors. If for instance, cheesecake is popular in one area but not in another, the manufacturers will know the exact ingredients of sugar, fat and salt to put into the cake that guarantee sales and repeat sales. The same goes for colas, fast foods and other junk food.

Focusing on cheesecake, cheesecake is manufactured with the correct ratio of sugar, fat and salt to make it desirable to eat. To give you some idea, and if you like cheesecake, in being offered or buying a cheesecake, you will almost be able to taste it while you are purchasing the product. When eating it, you would have scarcely finished one mouthful before putting the next fork full of cake into your mouth.

- First, seeing a portion of cheesecake will visually stimulate the tastebuds and receptors in your mouth – you have a desire to eat the cake.

- Secondly, you will cut a piece and pass it over your lips. You may even start to salivate.

- Once past your lips it touches your tongue, you feel the sensation of the collection of flavours burst; this stimulates your mouth senses. This sends the sensation of pleasure of sugar, fat and salt, through your neurotransmitters along your neuron pathways which spark your synapse system allowing the message of pleasure to rapidly reach your brain. Your memory makes a record of the way you feel and the pleasure you experience. Your mind is also in on the journey of satisfaction and pleasure. All of this information happens in a nanosecond or microsecond. Your 'pleasure centre' now wants more and then more.

The food manufacturers of the world spend a great deal of money ensuring that the 'bliss point' hits the right taste buds when a product is eaten.

The sweetness of sugar in its natural state is a very desirable food. Natural fat our body knows is good for us and within every living cell in our body there is a tiny amount of salt. So, for us to want or to crave the foods that have the 'bliss point' is a natural instinct. Karin Allen, PhD a professor of food science at Utah State University says,

*'In other words, it's a precise ratio, or formation, or concentration of certain nutrients the body is programmed to seek out and like (meaning fat, salt and sugar, which were key to survival in prehistoric times), combined in such a way as to make a food highly palatable.'[30]*

Howard Moskowitz is noted for his identification and development of the 'bliss point' in food. His research on Prego spaghetti sauce revealed a significant customer preference for an extra chunky product with an optimisation of sugar, salt and fat.

---

[30] https://www.youtube.com

There are many 'bliss points' that relate to different people and to different foods. It is however, the masses of people eating large quantities of processed food that contain the 'bliss point' that contribute to the damage of people's health, the obesity problem in the world and to the bad eating habits created through the lack of education from both the manufacturers of processed food, fast food chains and the education system itself.

**The devil's persuasion**

## The Devil in Sugar

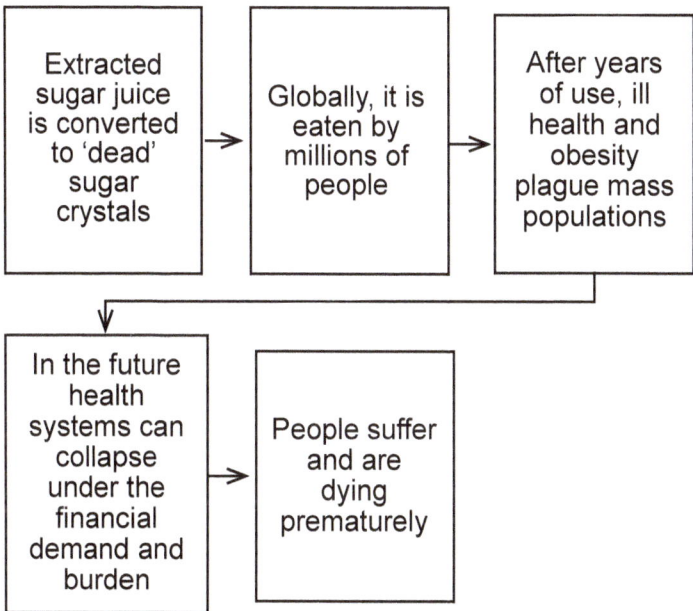

```
┌─────────────────┐     ┌─────────────────┐     ┌─────────────────┐
│ Extracted       │     │ Globally, it is │     │ After years     │
│ sugar juice     │     │ eaten by        │     │ of use, ill     │
│ is converted    │ ──> │ millions of     │ ──> │ health and      │
│ to 'dead'       │     │ people          │     │ obesity         │
│ sugar           │     │                 │     │ plague mass     │
│ crystals        │     │                 │     │ populations     │
└─────────────────┘     └─────────────────┘     └─────────────────┘
        │                                                 │
        └─────────────────────┬───────────────────────────┘
                              ▼
┌─────────────────┐     ┌─────────────────┐
│ In the future   │     │ People suffer   │
│ health          │     │ and are         │
│ systems can     │ ──> │ dying           │
│ collapse        │     │ prematurely     │
│ under the       │     │                 │
│ financial       │     │                 │
│ demand and      │     │                 │
│ burden          │     │                 │
└─────────────────┘     └─────────────────┘
```

**Your Notes**

...................................................................................................
...................................................................................................
...................................................................................................
...................................................................................................
...................................................................................................
...................................................................................................
...................................................................................................
...................................................................................................
...................................................................................................
...................................................................................................
...................................................................................................
...................................................................................................
...................................................................................................
...................................................................................................
...................................................................................................
...................................................................................................
...................................................................................................
...................................................................................................

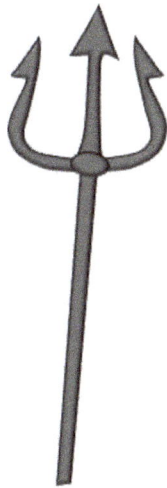

# Devils in Our Food

# Chapter Two ~ Fats
## The devil of trans-fat

The human body needs good fat. Fat, also known as triglyceride[31], cannot be taken from your body it needs to come from the food you eat. Fat like so many other foods needs to be eaten in moderation.

In Chapter One, I briefly spoke of molecules. Good fat or triglycerides also contain molecules. Good molecules are needed to allow your small intestine to continue to digest or mulch the food you eat and to pass the goodness through the intestine wall and into your blood stream. That then circulates through your body including your brain. The remains of the mulched food are sent into the large intestine where they are eventually excreted as waste.

Good fat molecules give your body energy and are important to maintain healthy skin, hair and organs. Your brain also requires a certain amount of good fat molecules, not too much, just enough. Fat also absorbs vitamins A, D, E and K; these are fat soluble vitamins. Your fat cells or molecules help to insulate your body to keep it warm, and in times of stress, because of the fat protective layer, helps to support your immune system.

Fats from your good food are called linoleic[32] and linolenic acid. These acids are essential because your

---

[31] Triglycerides are the main constituents of natural fats and oils.
[32] Is an omega-6 polyunsaturated fatty acid. Is essential for all humans and must be obtained through their diet.

body cannot work without them. They allow your blood to clot, help to control inflammation and support your brain in its working and development. This is why it's so important that babies, toddlers and children have the right type and amount of good fat in their diet.

Fats are made up of saturated and unsaturated fatty acids. Whether a fat is saturated or unsaturated will depend on how much acid the fat contains.

## Saturated fats – low density-lipoprotein or (LDL)

Saturated fats raise your low-density lipoproteins (LDL) this raises your cholesterol levels. This is also known as 'bad' fat. If your cholesterol levels are too high you are depositing fat within your arteries. By cholesterol forming in the arteries, it lessens the blood flow throughout your body. Fat can also deposit itself on your blood vessels; this in turn can harden and will lessen the oxygen levels delivered to your heart, brain and lungs. Eating food high in 'bad' LDL is a devil in your food and contributes nothing to your wellbeing, and long life. It will contribute to your ill health, pain, suffering and death.

## Unsaturated fats – high-density lipoprotein or (HDL)

Unsaturated fats contribute to high-density lipoprotein (HDL) and are 'good' and beneficial because they help to remove the LDL from your arteries and blood vessels and help to keep you healthy.

## Trans-fats

There are two types of good *trans-fat*s within food. The first are the *trans-fat*s that naturally occur in plants as they grow. The second *trans-fat*s are found in ruminant meat from cows, sheep and goats and in dairy products. These *trans-fat*s are natural and do not harm us if eaten in their natural state. The *trans*-fat I am speaking of in this book are the *trans-fat*s that are artificially manipulated and put into the food that is sold in supermarkets, fast food chains and other food outlets. These *trans-fat*s are **devils** in disguise and are found in 40 percent or more of the products on the supermarket shelves, in takeaway food outlets and small corner shops. *Trans-fat* **devils** hide in:

- **Snacks**: potato chips of many flavours; some pre-cooked and pre-prepared popcorn including microwavable popcorn, tortilla pancakes, manufactured French fries, chips, and corn chips.

- **Baked foods including**: cakes, biscuits and crackers (sweet and unsweetened), pies, frosting on unfrozen bought cakes including Danish pastries and biscuits and in commercially bought vegetable shortening.

- **Creamers and margarine**: non-dairy coffee creamers, margarines and some commercially produced bought foods containing creamers and margarine.

- **Commercially produced frozen pastry and dough**: frozen cakes of many types, tarts containing jam, apple and other fillings; sausage rolls including meat pies, commercially bought dough, pastry, pizza and doughnuts. *Trans-fat*s in doughnuts are one of the worst offending **devils** when it comes to the commercial manufacturing of food. They can contain up to 50 percent of *trans-fat* as part of their ingredients.

- **Commercially manufactured and cooked food:** deep fried fast foods cooked in *trans-fat*s in deep fryers and bought at outlets include: fish and chips, pie and chips, doughnuts, hash browns and chicken nuggets. When a *trans*-fat is used in cooking oil, it allows a longer shelf life and doesn't need to be changed or renewed as often.

- **Chocolate:** manufacturers of chocolate use *trans-fat*s in their production. Even expensive brands contain *trans-fat*s. *Trans-fat* allow the chocolate bar to be sold as a bar of chocolate otherwise, we would probably buy the chocolate in a bottle and drink it as a drink! That said, the *trans*-fat in a chocolate bar is doing no good to your health and wellbeing.

*Trans-fat*s or *trans*-fatty acids are considered, by many health practitioners, to be the worst type of fat we can eat; as previously mentioned, '*trans-fat*s raise your **'bad'** LDL cholesterol and lower the **'good'** HDL cholesterol resulting in poor health.'

*Trans-fat*s encourage the onset of heart disease, stroke, Diabetes Type 2, and other diseases and lead to an early death.

**The devils in *trans*-fats**

So what is a *trans*-fat and why is the medical profession and some governments around the world (not including Australia[33]), taking a long hard look at the way our food is prepared by large food corporations and manufacturers?

Most of the oils from the list below, when they are naturally distilled are healthy to have in our diets.

*Trans-fat* oils are manipulated through the process of hydrogenation[34]. Hydrogenation allows oils to be used in mass production; this causes the damage to our health.

Oils naturally extracted (always check extraction processes or methods) are:

- Olive
- Sunflower
- Coconut
- Safflower
- Sesame
- Grape seed
- Nuts including peanuts
- Soya bean
- Almond
- Walnuts and
- Palm kernel oil.

---

[33]Under Australian food law, manufacturers do not have to list *trans-fat* on the nutrition information panel of food products.
[34] Hydrogen is pumped into heating of hot oil which changes the molecular structure of the oil.

**Oils to avoid:**

The following oils are plant extracted but they are also not good for our health. They may also be hydrogenated.

**Avoid:**

- **Palm**
- **Rapeseed and**
- **Cotton oils**

**Hydrogenation and *trans-fat***

*Trans-fat*s are formed through industrial processes that pump hydrogen molecules into heated vegetable oils. A molecular reaction takes place by the insertion of either: **nickel**, **palladium** or **platinum** rods into heated or heating oil.

(In my research the type of metal rods were not identified nor were the number of metal rods used in each process to create *trans-fat*s).

The heat combined with the metal rod insertion changes the position of the hydrogen atom. The process of hydrogenation allows a liquid to become a solid. The procedure of hydrogenation changes the chemical structure of the oil. The solidification of the oil makes it easier for the spreading of butter and commercially made spreads. Once used in the cooking process, *trans-fat*s allows supermarkets, fast food outlets and highway food services to keep food sitting on the shelves for longer periods of time.

**Palm oil**

Palm oil is used widely in the production of cooking manufactured and processed foods. Palm oil is cheaper to produce and meets the demand for food oils in the fast food, fast food chain industries. Palm oil is also used in many supermarket products including: cakes, biscuits, chips and corn chips, sausage rolls, pies both sweet and savoury and other mass produced pastry products. As you go through the names below, some with their additive number will re-appear in Chapter Four.

**Other names given to palm oil**

- Acetic and fatty acid esters of glycerol (472a/e472a)
- Aluminium stearate
- Aluminium, calcium, sodium, magnesium salts of fatty acids (470/e470a; e470b)
- Ammonium laureth sulphate
- Ammonium lauryl sulphate
- Arachamide mea
- Ascorbyl palmitate
- Ascorbyl palmitate (304)
- Azelaic acid
- Butyl stearate
- Calcium lactylate
- Calcium oleyl lactylate
- Calcium stearate
- Calcium stearoyl lactylate (482/e482)
- Capric triglyceride
- Caprylic acid
- Caprylic triglyceride
- Caprylic/capric triglyceride
- Caprylic/capric/stearic triglyceride
- Capryloyl glycine
- Caprylyl glycol
- Ceteareth (2-100)

- Cetearyl alcohol
- Cetearyl ethylhexanote
- Cutter substitute (cbs)
- Cetearyl glucoside
- Cetearyl isononanoate
- Ceteth-20
- Ceteth-24
- Cetyl acetate
- Cetyl alcohol
- Cetyl ethylhexanoate
- Cetyl hydroxyethylcellulose
- Cetyl lactate
- Cetyl octanoate
- Cetyl palmitate
- Cetyl ricinoleate
- Citric and fatty acid esters of glycerol (472c/e472c)
- Cocoa butter equivalent (cbe)
- Cocoa
- Cecyl oleate
- Diacetyltartaric and fatty acid esters of glycerol (472e/e472e)
- Dilinoleic acid
- Disodium lauryl sulfosuccinate
- Distilled monoglyceride palm
- Elaeis guineensis oil
- Emulsier 422, 430-36, 470-8, 481-483, 493-5
- Epoxidized palm oil (uv cured coatings)
- Ethyl lauroyl arginate (243)
- Ethylene glycol monostearate
- Ethylhexyl hydroxystearate
- Ethylhexyl palmitate
- Ethylhexyl stearate
- Ethylhexylglycerin
- Glycerin
- Glycerin or glycerol (442)
- Glyceryl distearate
- Glyceryl laurate
- Glyceryl monostearate
- Glyceryl myristate
- Glyceryl oleate

- Glyceryl polymethacrylate
- Glyceryl stearate
- Glyceryl stearate se
- Glycol distearate
- Glycol stearate
- Guineesis (palm)
- Hexadecylic
- Hexyl laurate
- Hexyldecanol
- Hydrogenated palm glycerides
- Isopropyl isostearate
- Isopropyl palmitate
- Isopropyl titanium triisostearate
- Isostearamide dea
- Isostearate dea
- Isostearic acid
- Isostearic acid
- Isostearyl alcohol
- Lactic and fatty acid easters of glycerol (472b/e472b)
- Lauramide dea
- Lauramide mea
- Lauramine oxide
- Laureth
- Lauric acid lauroyl sarcosine
- Lauryl betaine
- Lauryl lactate
- Lauryl glucoside (from palm)
- Lauryl pyrrolidone
- Linoleic acid
- Magnesium myristate
- Magnesium stearate
- Mixed tartaric, acetic and fatty acid esters of glycerol (472f/e472f )
- Mono-and- di-glycerides of fatty acids (471/e471)
- Myristate
- Myristic acid
- Myristic cetrimonium chloride acid
- Myristoyl
- Myristyl alcohol

- Myristyl myristate
- Medium chain triglycerides (mcts)
- Octyl palmitate
- Octyl stearate
- Octyldodecyl myristate
- Octyldodecyl stearoyl stearate
- Oleamide mipa
- Oleic acid
- Oleyl betaine
- Palm fruit oil
- Palm kernel oil
- Palm oil
- Palm olein
- Palm stearine
- Palmate
- Palmitate
- Palmitic acid
- Palmitamidopropyltrimonium chloride
- Palmitoyl myristyl serinate
- Palmitoyl oxostearamide
- Palmitoyl oligopeptide
- Palmitoyl tetrapeptide-3
- Peg-100 stearate
- Palmityl alcohol
- Retinyl palmitate
- Red palm oil
- Saponified elaeis guineensis
- Saturated fatty acid
- Sleareth
- Sles
- Sls
- Sodium alkyl sulfate
- Sodium cetearyl sulphate
- Sodium cocoyl glycinate
- Sodium cocoyl isethionate
- Sodium dodecylbenzenesulfonate
- Sodium dodecyl sulphate (sds or nads)
- Sodium isostearoyl lactylaye
- Sodium lactylate; sodium oleyl lactylate; sodium
- Stearoyl lactylate

- Sodium laurate
- Sodium laurel
- Sodium laureth sulfate
- Sodium laureth 1 sulphate
- Sodium laureth 2 sulphate
- Sodium laureth 3 sulphate
- Sodium laureth-13 carboxylate
- Sodium lauroyl lactylate
- Sodium lauryl
- Sodium lauryl ether sulphate
- Sodium lauryl glucose carboxylate
- Sodium lauryl lactylate/sulphate
- Sodium lauryl sulfoacetate
- Sodium lauroyl sarcosinate
- Sodium methyl cocoyl taurate
- Sodium myristate
- Sodium palm kernelate
- Sodium plam kerneloyl isethionate
- Sodium plamate
- Sodium plamitate
- Sodium polyartlsulfonate
- Sodium stearate
- Sodium stearoyl fumarate
- Sodium stearoyl glutamate
- Sodium stearoyl lactylate
- Sodium trideceth sulphate
- Solubiliser ps20
- Sorbitan caprylate
- Sorbitan cocoate
- Sorbitan diisostearate
- Sorbitan distearate
- Sorbitan ester
- Sorbitan isotearate
- Sorbitan laurate
- Sorbitan monoglyceride
- Sorbitan monolaurate
- Sorbitan monopalmitate
- Sorbitan monostearate (491)
- Sorbitan oleate
- Sorbitan olivate
- Sorbitan palmitate

- Sorbitan sesquioleate
- Sorbitan trioleate
- Sorbitan tristearate
- Sorbitan tristearate (492)
- Sorbitan triglyceride
- Stearalkonium chloride
- Stearalkonium hectorite
- Stearamide mea
- Stearamidopropyl dimethylamine
- Steareth-2
- Steareth-7
- Steareth-10
- Steareth-20
- Steareth-21
- Stearic acid
- Stearic acid or fatty acid (570)
- Stearoyl sarcosine
- Stearyl alcohol
- Stearyl dimethicone
- Stearyl heptanoate
- Stearyl tartarate
- Stearyltrimetylammonium chloride
- Stearoyl lactic acid
- Stearoyl sarcosine
- Steartrimonium chloride
- Succinylated monoglycerides
- Sucrose esters of fatty acids
- Sucrose stearate
- Sucroseesters of fatty acids
- Sulphonated methyl esters
- Surfactant ccg
- taxanomic
- Tea-lauryl sulphate
- Tea-stearate
- Tetradecyloctadecyl myristate
- Tmp esters
- Tocotrienols (vitamin e)
- Tocopherols (vitamin e)
- Tocopheryl linoleat
- Triacetin
- Triacetin (1518)

- Tribehenin
- Tricaprylin
- Tridecyl myristate
- Tristearin
- Veg-emulse
- Vegetable emulsifier
- Vegetable glycerin
- Vegetable oil
- Vitamin a palmitate
- Yeast with 491
- Yeast powder with 491
- Zinc idne laureth
- Zinc myristate
- Zinc stearate[35]

Once commodities like palm oil disperse into the supply and food chain, the pathways to the final product are often complex and obscured. From the plantation to the supermarket shelf or fast food chain outlet, there could be a number of multiple and complex stages of production to the original palm kernel or palm oil that results in the ingredient not necessarily having to be listed as 'palm oil'.

## Coconut oil hidden devil or not?

From the Heart Foundation: *'You've probably seen claims about coconut oil being a healthy food, and perhaps even a superfood. Coconut oil is 92 percent saturated fat, and recent reviews of evidence show that coconut oil consumption raises your total blood cholesterol (both good HDL and bad LDL cholesterol and increases your risk of heart disease. The research suggests coconut oil may be better than butter in how*

---

[35] https://orangutanalliance.org

*it affects blood cholesterol, but it's not as good as other plant oils like olive and canola oil.*[36]

## Further research on coconut oil – the experiment

Dr. Michael Mosley of the television program, Trust Me I'm A Doctor and two researchers: Professor Kay-Tee Khaw and Professor Nita Forouhi from the University of Cambridge in the United Kingdom conducted an experiment to see if coconut oil was either **good** or **bad** to have in the diet. One hundred volunteers, over the age of 50 years, would have their cholesterol levels tested after eating coconut oil, when compared to other fats, in their diets.

The volunteers were split into three groups.

Every day, for four weeks, the volunteers added one of three fats to their diets.

*'Group 1 had 50 grams of coconut oil a day.*
*Group 2 had 50 grams of olive oil a day and*
*Group 3 ate 50 grams of butter a day.'*

The results of the experiment were as follows:

*'For LDL cholesterol, associated with an increased risk of heart disease:*

*For butter, study participants had an average increase in LDL cholesterol by 0.3 millimoles per litre, representing a rise of around 10 percent. The increased risk to heart health reverted back once the regime was stopped.*

---

[36] https://www.heartfoundation.org.au

*For olive oil, there was a very small average reduction which was not statistically significant. This means there was essentially no difference in LDL cholesterol with participants on the olive oil diet.*

*For coconut oil, LDL cholesterol decreased by 0.09 millimoles per litre. This was not statistically significant, so overall results show there was no increase in LDL cholesterol for the coconut oil group.* [37]

The research identified a rise in both the LDL and HDL when coconut oil was ingested. However, because coconut oil is rich in lauric acid,[38] coconut oil may have other health advantages.

The researchers concluded: *'One explanation for the results is that coconut oil is rich in lauric acid, which may be processed in the body differently...'*[39]

Accordingly, lauric acid increases total serum cholesterol more than any other fatty acids but most of the increase is made possible by an increase in high-density lipoprotein (HDL) (the good blood cholesterol).

The Heart foundation has also warned about eating butter.

Butter is made up of 50 percent of saturated fat with 4 percent of *trans-fats*. Even in the latest television documentaries, health gurus have promoted eating butter over any of the supermarket mass sold margarines.

---

[37] https://www.bbc.co.uk

[38] Found in human breast milk, cows' and goats' milk.

[39] Prof Kay-Tee Khaw www.phpc.cam.ac.uk, Prof Nita Forouhi www.mrc-epid.cam.ac.uk

Accordingly, olive oil, avocados, nut butter made from almonds or tahina are natural butters and provide your body with unsaturated fats, minimal saturated fats and no *trans-fats*.

## *Trans-fats* – the development of the devil

Understanding how and what a *trans*-fat is will allow people to become aware of the modification and adaption to our food that manufacturers use to satisfy their profit margins!

*Trans-fat*ty acids or *trans-fats* are a form of saturated fat used widely in the processed food industry. Unlike unsaturated fat, *trans-fat* to your body, is like eating candle wax. Your body cannot process it, the gut will reject it. This fat then has nowhere to go other than to your arteries.

*Trans-fat* is a manmade product first developed in 1809 by Paul Sabatier a Nobel prize winner for his work in Chemistry. In 1901, Wilhelm Normann, a German chemist showed that liquid oils could be hydrogenated and patented the process in 1902. Normann's process of hydrogenation showed that whale and fish oil could be stabilised and used for human consumption.

*Trans-fats* have been in continuous use, modified and in large scale food processing and production since that time.

## Molecules and how they work?

a) A fat molecule is made up of a glycerol head and
   three fatty acid tails each of which is a hydrogen and
   carbon chain.

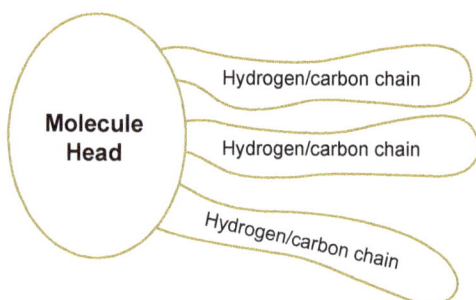

Each molecule is so small it could take 100 million of
them to make an inch. They cannot be seen with the
naked eye.

Each tail attached to the head of the molecule contains
a combination of letters and numbers which form
hydrocarbon and carbon chains.

The enlarged diagram on this page shows the working
components of a molecule.

## Saturated fat

b)

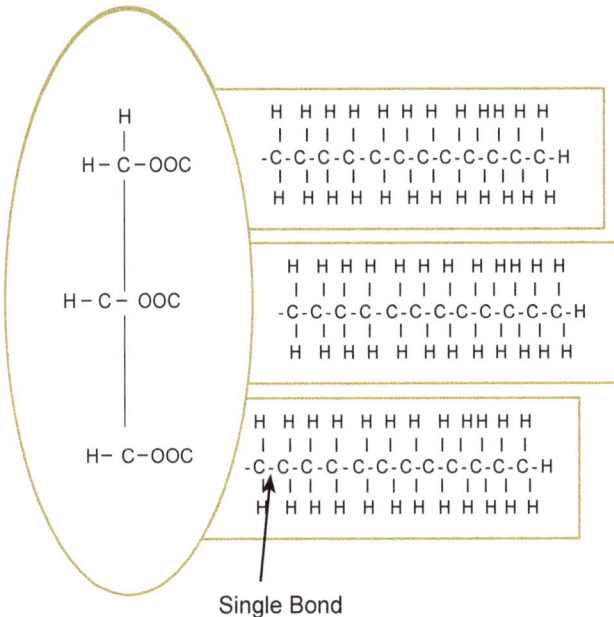

```
                    H  H H H  H H H  H HH H H
                    |  | | |  | | |  | || | |
H – C – OOC       -C-C-C-C -C-C-C-C-C-C-C-C-H
                    |  | | |  | | |  | | | | |
                    H  H H H  H H H  H H H H H

                    H  H H H  H H H  H HH H H
                    |  | | |  | | |  | || | |
H – C – OOC       -C-C-C-C -C-C-C-C-C-C-C-C-H
                    |  | | |  | | |  | | | | |
                    H  H H H  H H H  H H H H H

                    H  H HH  H H H  H HH H H
                    |  | | |  | | |  | || | |
H – C – OOC       -C-C-C-C -C-C-C-C-C-C-C-C-H
                    |  | | |  | | |  | | | | |
                    H  H H H  H H H  H H H H H
```

Single Bond

'C' in the above diagram stands for carbon atom and 'H' for hydrogen. When all of the carbons (C) are bound to hydrogen (H), within a straight chain and are connected by a single bond they are said to be saturated. Due to their straight tails they are compact and hard at room temperature. To give you an example, a slab of butter or margarine would be a saturated fat.

A fat molecule made entirely of fatty acids is a saturated fat.

## Unsaturated fat

On the other hand, when a hydrocarbon chain has fewer hydrogen atoms, it is said to be unsaturated.

c)

### Fewer hydrogen atoms

```
H   H H   H   H          H  H H  H   H
|   | |   |   |   |   |   |  | |  |   |
-C -C -C -C  -C -C -C -C  -C -C -C -C- H
|   | |   |   |   |   |   |  |  |   |  |
H   H H   H   H   H H   H  H  H  H H  H
```

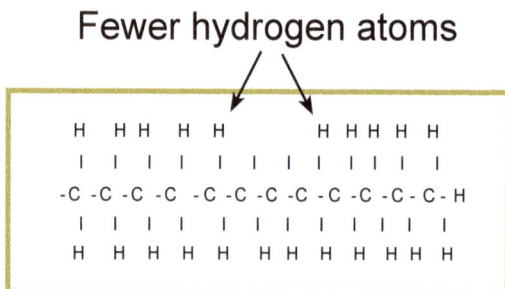

Instead of binding to a maximum number of hydrogen atoms some carbon atoms bind to each other creating a double bond.

d)

### Double bond

```
H   H H  H    H          H  H H  H  H
|   | |  |    |   |   |   |  | |  |  |
-C - C - C - C  -C - C = C - C -C - C -C- C- H
|   | |  |    |   |   |   |  |  |  |   |
H   H H  H    H   H H   H  H  H  H H  H
```

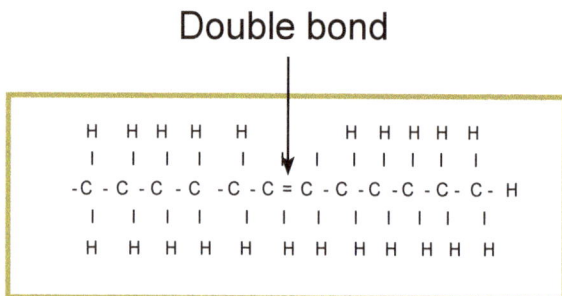

The double bond between carbons makes them less compact or hard at room temperature therefore, they are not as fluid as seen in cooking oils.

You can see how one of the tail's bend in a mono[40] unsaturated molecule. A fat liquid that contains only one double bond is a mono-unsaturated fat.

e)

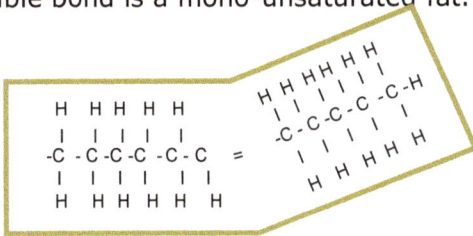

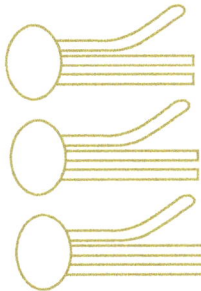

Mono unsaturated fat

A molecule that has many double bonds with the tails separate and fluid create poly unsaturated fat.

f)

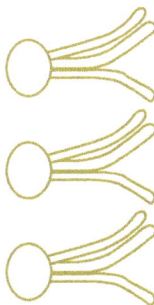

Poly unsaturated fat

---

Many dietary fats provide fatty acids for synthesis within the cell membrane and are a vital component for all animal cells including human cells.

g)

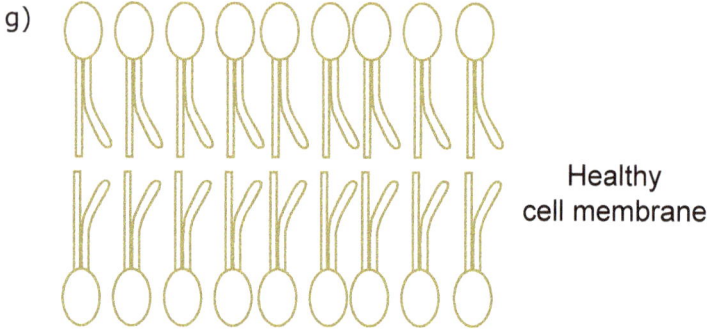

Healthy
cell membrane

The gaps in unsaturated fatty acids maintain flexibility and contribute to a healthy cell membrane allowing for movement and cellular signalling.

h)

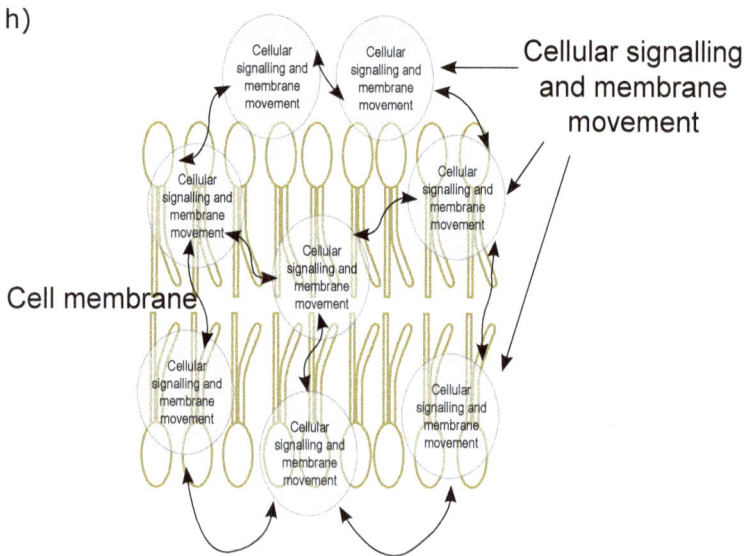

Cellular signalling and membrane movement

Cell membrane

Healthy fats are needed for optimal structure of the membrane. However, too much saturated fat, which is now the case in many Western, Asian and world diets, make the membranes rigid and hard and hinder cellular receptiveness and movement.

i)

## Optimal saturated/unsaturated fat ratio

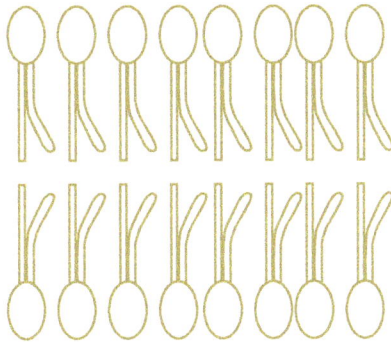

Too much saturated fat leads to slowness of cell signalling and the lack of fluidity within the membrane/s.

Membrane fluidity is most important in the nervous system where neuronal responsiveness requires extremely fast transaction and communication. Slowness in responding to situations when driving a vehicle, farm equipment, aircraft, operating machinery or any situation where a quick response is needed may show there is slowness in your cell signalling and membrane movement. This may also indicate a build-up of cholesterol in your system.

When you are thinking on your feet, you feel good, feel healthy and are ready for the next challenge in life. If this is not the case, your diet may be holding you back.

Too much saturated fat will make you feel unwell. Your brain does not work as it did and you are feeling it's all too much. Please now look at the food you're eating and how much processed food you're putting into your body's system.

Remember, you don't have taste buds in your stomach only in your mouth and it's your brain's 'pleasure centre' in combination with the ghrelin cells[41] released from your gut area that may be demanding more high cholesterol food. Over time, because you weren't aware of *trans-fat*s, you may have become a 'junk food junkie!'

Too much saturated fat will make you feel sick.

j)                  Too much saturated fat

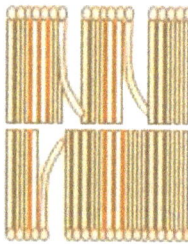

The tails of the majority of
molecules are pushed
together restricting cellular
signalling and membrane
movement

---

[41] Ghrelin is a hormone produced in the pancreas and stomach. It's also known as the 'hunger hormone'

When the molecules in your brain and system are pushed together as in diagram (j), your comprehension of events and situations may be slow.

A combination of good saturated and unsaturated fatty acids is required to keep the myelin[42] sheaf, the insulation material that wraps around axons of the neurons, which helps to keep them healthy. Axons and neurons are in your brain and run down your spine connecting to the gut. Myelin speeds up the conduction of electrical signals from your senses to your brain and the reactions you have or need to take.

The body is capable of synthesizing all of the oil and fatty acids it needs with the exception of essential fatty acids which must be obtained from your diet which include:

- Polyunsaturated fats
- Omega 3 and 6 foods.

**Polyunsaturated fat include:**

- o Corn
- o Flax
- o Oatmeal
- o Walnuts.

Omega 3 and 6 should be taken in moderation.

**Omega 3 foods include:**

- o Soybeans
- o Cold-pressed olive oil

---

[42] A fatty white substance that protects the axons of some nerve cells.

- Pumpkin seeds
- Mackerel
- Pecan nuts
- Cod liver oil
- Flax seed
- Salmon
- Walnuts and
- Chia seeds.

**Omega 6 foods include:**

- Wheat germ
- Sunflower oil
- Safflower oil
- Poppy seed
- Walnut oil
- Corn oil
- Some cotton seed oil
- Soybean oil and sesame oil.

These oils need to be uncontaminated and free of hydrogenation.

### *Trans-fat* – the unhealthy, saturated fat

*Trans-fat*, the lurking devil should be avoided.

I have spoken about the molecules in our foods on the previous pages; the story has been leading up to this point.

Before going to the story of *trans*-fat, let's take a step backwards and again look at LDL and HDL, these cholesterol levels were first mentioned on page 59. When not understanding the differences between unsaturated fat, saturated fat and *trans-fat*s, the supermarket products and their labelling become a minefield of confusion. I too have been so confused about product labelling that is just one of the reasons I have decided to write this book.

## Fats Identified

k) **Unsaturated Fat molecule**  **Saturated Fat molecule**  *Trans Fat molecule*

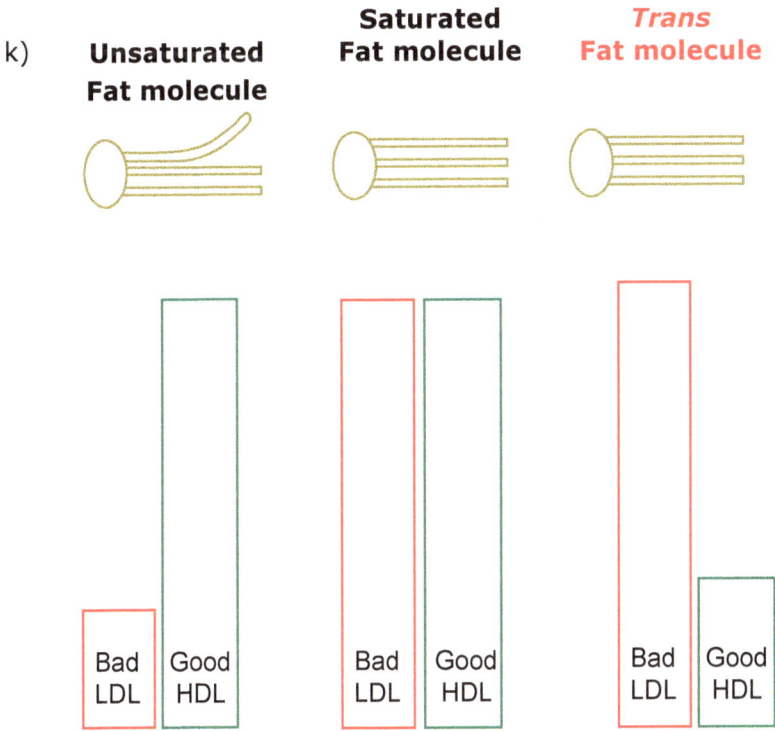

In the above:

- Unsaturated fat allows the good cholesterol to rise and keeps you healthy
- Saturated fat raises both your good and bad cholesterol. Please also refer to the BBC – the coconut oil research project on page 71.

- *Trans-fat* raises your bad cholesterol while lowering your good cholesterol.

Each tail of the molecule carries information about hydrogen and carbon atoms. It's the chemistry in the tails of the molecules that make fat either good or bad.

## Unsaturated fat and *trans*-fat

In general unsaturated fats are good for you. They reduce the possibility of heart disease by raising the good HDL cholesterol. They also reduce the bad cholesterol or LDL. Not all unsaturated fats are equal. In some fresh foods, natural *trans*-fat are also known as an unsaturated fat. It's hydrogenated, please remember it's the immersion of either nickel, palladium or platinum rods into heated oil, that creates a commercial *trans*-fat.

Because of the processing, *Trans*-fat is the unhealthiest of all fats. The information in the tail of the molecule is what makes the difference to a 'good' or 'bad' fat.

When the information in the tail is changed and becomes a 'double bond'. A double-bond can give rise to two configurations:

a) a semi-curved tail in the carbon structure as in unsaturated fat, or
b) a straight tail in the carbon structure of a *trans*-fat.

This transformation leads to two different types of fat. *Cis* is when the hydrogen atoms are on the same side of the bond. Please see diagram I below.

*Cis* is contained within unsaturated fat.

### *Cis* hydrogen atoms

l)

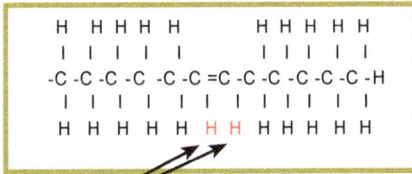

*Cis* is when the hydrogen atoms
are *on the same side of the bond*

The *Cis* double bond bends the fatty acid molecule and takes on the shape of a semi-curve. A *Cis* double bond is within foods that are grown and produced by nature: plants that naturally grow and meat from naturally reared animals including: cow, lamb and goat and some dairy products. These foods, in their natural state, contain natural *trans-fats* that are digestible by the human gut. Our gut has the enzymes to break down this natural *trans-fat*.

### *Cis* hydrogen atom cells – double bond

m)

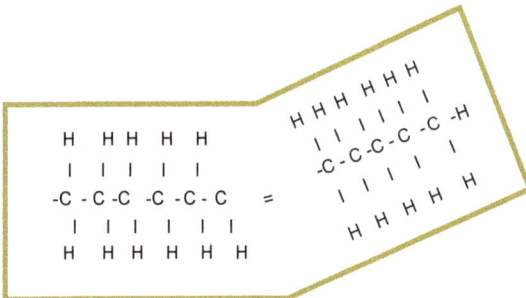

## Natural *Trans-fat*

A natural *trans*-fat is similar in structure to a saturated fat. It's important to know, *trans-fat*s are rare in nature, apart from the few previously mentioned: plants, in small numbers and in meat which include: cows, sheep, goats and some dairy foods.

Man-made *trans*-fat have a different chemical formation in hydrogen atoms. It is this difference that causes:

- Obesity
- Many health problems and sickness
- Cholesterol related illnesses
- Diabetes Type 2 and has
- Detrimental effects on blood vessels.

*Trans-fat*s are made by manipulation of the hydrogen atom. The hydrogen atom is on the opposite side of the carbon as seen in diagram (n) on the following page.

Foods containing *trans-fat*s will lower your **good HDL** and raise your **bad LDL**.

n)

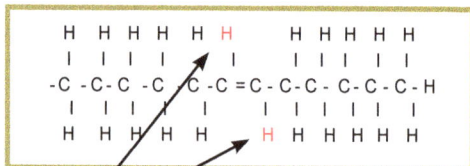

*Trans* is when the hydrogen atoms are on opposite sides of the molecule tail

86

## Effects of eating too much *trans-fat*

Eating hydrogenated *Trans*-fat leads to:

- Clogged arteries
- Heart disease raising the risk of heart attack
- Stroke and possibly
- Diabetes Type 2.

Food manufacturers, including bakeries prefer to add hydrogenated fats to their products. By this process:

- More texture is added to the product
- Shelf life is prolonged
- Spoiling is decreased and
- Production costs are reduced making food production cheaper and more affordable for mass market consumption.

## *Cis* vs *Trans* – partial hydrogenation

o)

Molecule head          Molecule head

$+H_2$ →

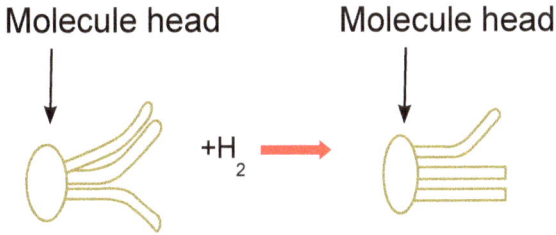

Unfortunately, partial hydrogenation also converts some of the *cis* hydrogen cells into *trans-fat*.

*Trans-fat*s are found mainly in partially hydrogenated, hydrogenated or modified oil products such as margarine. Hydrogenation turns oils into solid or semi-solid products. *Trans-fat*s are also found in some ice creams and in many foods for children. Always read the product label before you buy. For more information on molecular formation, please see Medical Media.com[43]

## A chemistry approach

Bringing the last eleven pages together – understanding *trans-fat*s. From edublogs.[44]

p)

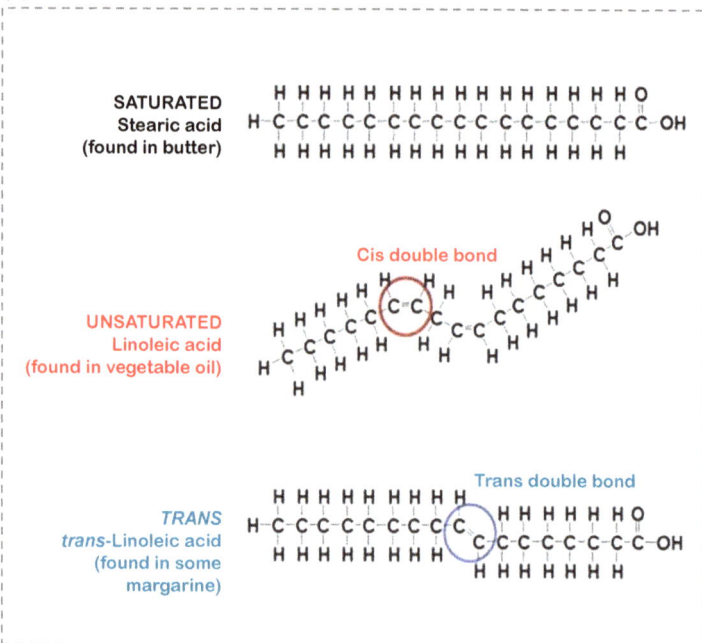

| | |
|---|---|
| **SATURATED** Stearic acid (found in butter) | Cis double bond |
| **UNSATURATED** Linoleic acid (found in vegetable oil) | |
| *TRANS* trans-Linoleic acid (found in some margarine) | Trans double bond |

---

[43] In recognition: www. Alila Medical Media . com
[44] In recognition: edublogs.org

### Trans-fat

Is a destructive ingredient put into many commercially produced and bought foods; we need to be vigilant and 'on our toes' if we are to be aware of the ingredients the food manufacturers put into their food products. We pay good money to buy good food. To date, much of the food bought does not justify the money paid.

### Trans-fat and your body

We were originally hunter gatherers and are programmed to like fat or oils. Simply put, fats were rare in the time of our ancient ancestors'. The animals they slaughtered weren't fat, if they were, they would be easy targets for their predators and survival rates would have been low.

Our ancestors were also lean and not conditioned to the abundance and easy access to over-sugared, over-processed, over cooked or hydrogenated food as we are today. I have previously mentioned '...our bodies do not have the required enzymes...' to break down trans-fats. Many unwanted or poison enzymes are left in the gut and stomach and result in unwanted belly fat, thigh fat, extra fat and possibly ill health.

The human body has taken thousands of years to reach its latest evolution. As previously said, 'We are equipped to eat food containing natural trans-fats which are produced naturally.' The journey of the destructive trans-fat is now in human evolution and we don't know what the outcome will be for future generations.

As I have previously mentioned, 'trans-fats are put into food to prolong shelf life, enhance texture' and to appeal to our eyes which then stimulates 'mouthfeel'. If addicted, we find the food cooked with *trans*-fat almost irresistible.

## Further brain research

The journey of the *trans*-fat doesn't stop once eaten. If you are fortunate, the end product is reduced by your gut enzymes and the residue is released through the end of your anus!

Some of those tiny *trans*-fat molecules, because they cannot pass through your system, may now be circulating within your body and more detrimentally, within your brain and other soft tissue areas.

Originally, we collected most of our meat and fish from their natural environments. We grew some of our plant food; some grew naturally on trees, in hedgerows, around coast lines such as seaweeds and, some grew randomly in fields from natural distribution by birds or insects. These foods were and are healthy for us to eat. *Trans-fat* on the other hand is not.

## *Trans-fat* and glia

Glia means 'glue' and is part of the chemistry of the brain, the central nervous system and the spinal cord. Glia also plays a role in the neurotransmission of synaptic connections. This means it helps to keep the information moving through your brain and allows you to make decisions, have assumptions, form ideas and take actions if needed.

In the brain, glia has four main functions:

1. Supply oxygen to nutrients and neurons
2. Surround neurons and hold them in place
3. Insulate one neuron from another
4. Destroy pathogens and remove dead neurons.

Some recent research on the role of *trans-fat*s and its penetration into the human brain should start to ring loud negative bells in your head.

As an educator, I study the topic of behaviour. Behaviour is an outcome of:

1. Past-experience (both good and bad)

2. How the information is processed from the senses of touching, hearing, seeing, feeling and experiencing (past or current situations)

3. The ideas *trans*mitted from the processing into thoughts and future actions. (The actions may be immediate or premeditated.) And lastly

4. The action/s finally takes place.

This synthesis of information can happen in a nanosecond of time and all is processed in your brain.

Processing information takes energy which is provided by the food you eat.

From research now being carried out by eminent scientists such as Andrew Koob and others, there is a positive link to *trans-fat*s and the detriment of memory or recall.

'*Trans-fats were most strongly linked to the worse memory, in young and middle-aged men, during their working and career-building years,*' said Beatrice A Golomb, M.D., PhD lead author and professor of medicine at the University of California-San Diego.[45]

We know that the formation of the hydrogen atom is changed through hydrogenation or partial hydrogenation of food oils. Food oils exist in most of the foods we eat and are almost unavoidable in most diets.

Professor Golomb has also identified that most '*trans-fat consumption has been linked to higher body weight, more aggression and heart disease.*'

Given this research, it would correlate with my own experiences and observational research of the young men I counselled and taught while working in the prison system in the United Kingdom. It would also answer some of the questions of 'Why?' children misbehave during lesson time and school time. It may also answer some of the questions of 'why?' has cyber bullying become so rampant in some of the school and education environments within Australia, America and the United Kingdom. Also on the rise is sexting[46].

Golomb's further research: '*Foods have different effects on oxidative stress and cell energy.*' said Professor Golomb.[47]

---

[45] https://www.golombresearchgroup.org
[46] Sexting is forwarding or receiving explicit messages, photographs or images sent through mobile phones.
[47] Golomb, Beatrice, Scientific Conferences & Meetings (November 2014).

## The human brain

For the human species to survive, the brain must be protected. The food conglomerates have had a *'field day'* since the end of the First and second World Wars.

Throughout the First and Second World Wars, food had been scarce and people were happy to be fed an affordable diet regardless of its illegitimate food value. Processed food was cheaper, easy to buy, prepare and serve up to families. Cooked, ready to eat food has been made convenient. Despite significant processing, it was and is still seen as easy and good to eat. With decades of eating 'junk food' we are now seeing the destructive outcomes of those years:

1. Obesity levels are higher than in human history
2. Heart disease is on the increase
3. There are more molecular disorders than previously recorded
4. Diabetes Type 2 is increasing
5. There's possibly brain damage for the future generations and
6. The debilitating effects of 'junk food' on young people causing blindness and deafness. Please refer to page 30, and the article in The Telegraph.

The fast food chains have caused **health havoc** by 'cashing in' on the processing hysteria that has taken place over the last 50 years, but now it's time to change our attitudes and actions when choosing the food we eat.

By functional design, a molecule is triangular in shape and three-dimensional; they are smaller than the full stop seen at the end this sentence.

Suzana Herculano-Houzel, PhD, Associate Professor of Psychology and Biological Science, Vanderbilt Brain Institute, Vanderbilt University, has established that the human brain consists of about 86 billion neurons. This number is considerably larger than in other primate brains. Though not confirmed Herculano-Houzel suggests: *'Our big brains are very costly. They use 25 percent of all the energy the body needs each day,'* she said. *'Cooking allowed us to overcome an energetic barrier that restricts the size of the brains of other primates.*[48]

## Your bodily system and *trans-fat*

Below, imagine this is a complete molecule of unsaturated fat, (enlarged idea). The head and tails are complete in the shape shown.

Molecules are complex arrangements of hydrogen and carbon atoms. For simplicity sake, the molecule below has been kept to a pyramid shape to allow for simple explanation.

## Molecule of unsaturated fat

q)

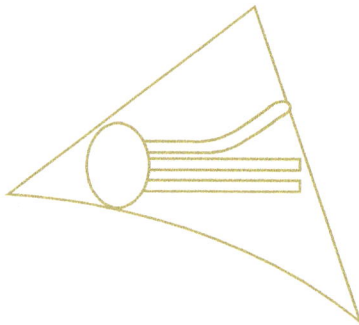

---

[48] https://news.vanderbilt.edu

When fluid, the shape resembles a half-moon. If you hold your hand in front of you, bend your index finger to form a half-moon shape, it will give you some idea of a healthy, unsaturated fat molecule profile.

Because of the shape, the molecule has room to move, this allows for cellular signalling and membrane movement.

Now let's take this idea a little further.

**A healthy adult human brain showing the molecule of unsaturated fat and healthy neuron and synapse connections**

The brain needs to stay functional and healthy. (Following on, in number order, from diagram 7, page 41).

8) Synapse sparks, healthy neuron connections, cellular signalling and membrane movement work together in a healthy brain

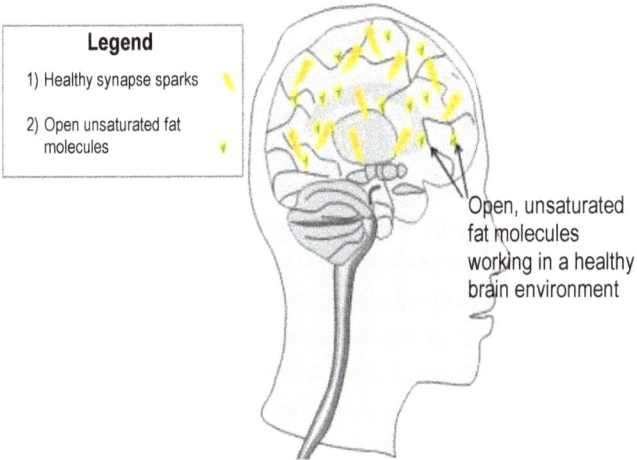

Legend

1) Healthy synapse sparks

2) Open unsaturated fat molecules

Open, unsaturated fat molecules working in a healthy brain environment

## Trans-fats and neuron connections

Given there are about 86 billion neurons inside your head, each neuron needs protection; it makes sense to eat a healthy diet which adds to this protection.

In Professor Golomb's research it was noted: 'We found that the higher the trans-fat consumption, the worse the memory performance, in younger adult ages, during key career building years.'

## Trans-fat again

In 3, in the Legend below, the dark colour, solid rectangle shape represents the tran- fat molecules and how they block free-flowing information in cellular signalling and membrane movement.

9)

Trans fats produce a flat, closed hard molecule

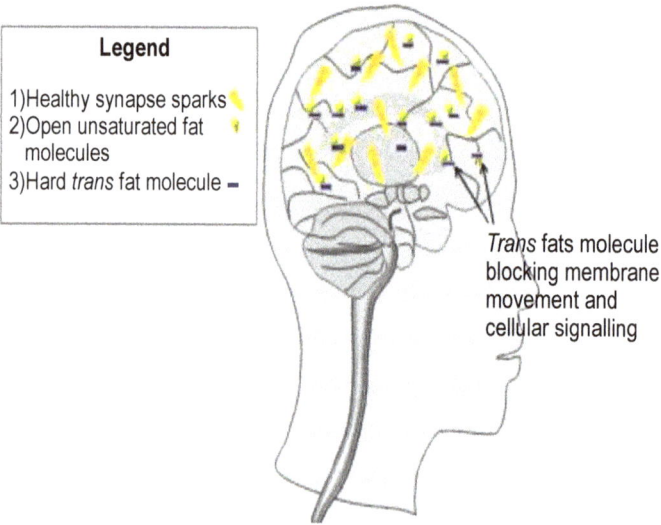

Legend

1)Healthy synapse sparks
2)Open unsaturated fat molecules
3)Hard trans fat molecule –

Trans fats molecule blocking membrane movement and cellular signalling

It is now becoming evident, eating an unhealthy diet will lead to illness. It could be suggested that a current diet high in *trans-fat*s, as in the diagram on the previous page shows, will lead to brain re-construction. The re-construction, like all evolutionary processes, will be done by the brain adapting to its own environment.

Re-construction may take generations. It may interfere with your DNA. Over thousands of generations and evolution, your brain has learnt to modify and adapt. Will it do the same to the *trans-fat*s in this world of processed food?

What we don't know at this point:

- Will *trans-fat*s cause disfigurement in and of the brain?
- Will *trans-fat*s cause physical limb or senses disfigurement in the next or future generations?
- It has possibly been a big contributor to youth blindness and deafness as seen on page 30, earlier in the book.

We simply have no idea of how changing the brain chemistry will change the DNA of the future generations. It seems extremely unfair to me to put this burden on our grandchildren and future great grandchildren.

Many scientific papers are now identifying the negative processes on health when food is prepared and cooked with oils that have been through the process of hydrogenation or partial hydrogenation.

**The human brain suffers**

As the mounting evidence is showing, regular eating of three *trans*-fat meals a day may do significant damage to the human brain, this research is ongoing. As research has shown, a *trans*-fat rich diet does nothing for the cognitive ability of the human being, it makes a person:

- Physically slow
- Sluggish
- Under active
- Angry
- Frustrated
- Lethargic and
- May lead to depression and
- Weight gain.

It is not clear at this point, whether the molecule of *trans-fat* stays within the brain or if the molecule can be removed by a person changing to a healthy diet.

The body and brain being of a forgiving nature, once the poison is stopped, may start to cleanse itself to become healthy and whole again. Recent experiments have suggested this may happen.

# The human brain under strain

10)

The brain under strain from *trans* fat molecule overload

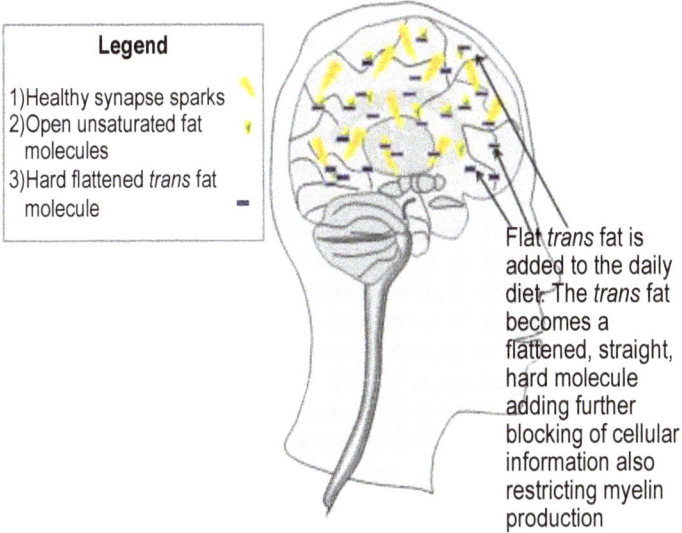

**Legend**

1) Healthy synapse sparks
2) Open unsaturated fat molecules
3) Hard flattened *trans* fat molecule

Flat *trans* fat is added to the daily diet. The *trans* fat becomes a flattened, straight, hard molecule adding further blocking of cellular information also restricting myelin production

The marketing of quick available food is targeting not only young people but also to the 'grey' generation.

In a television advertisement seen over Christmas 2018, the main characters were older, affluent Australians seen lounging and enjoying a poolside party. The crescendo to the advertisement was a glamorous, older woman dressed in up-market swim wear walking around the pool offering pieces of cooked, crumbed chicken. At that point, a senior, fit, male model walks into the picture wearing a pair of red and white stripped budgie smugglers and an expensive silk dressing gown. On seeing the male, the woman's eyes tell the story: her mouth falls open, her eyes light up as she offers him a piece of 'hot' crumbed chicken...! Close of advertisement.

Such advertising may lure that age group to buy. This group may want to live the fantasy seen in the advertisement. It may also lure them to take their grandchildren to the closest fast food outlet creating another memory connection in a younger generation!

Of course, a now and again outing is good for anyone but it's the regularity and quantity of *trans-fat*s that cause health problems.

## Children's brains and *trans-fat*s

If the previous pages have not frightened you to death, this piece of information will shake you up. As a parent, I only wanted the best for my children. The best meant in everything I did for them including the food they had to eat.

For the most part, all parents want the best outcome for their children and family. A child's brain takes many years to mature, in fact up to the age of 25 a young person's brain goes through infancy, adolescence or puberty and then into maturity. Over this time, neurotransmitters, synapse placement and the physical development of the brain all take place.

When a child or adult eats food, junk or otherwise, it will take between 24 to 72 hours for the food to pass out through the anus opening. As the child chews, glands in the mouth release a saliva containing enzymes, these help to breakdown the solid food matter. When the food is swallowed, it travels down the oesophagus. The oesophagus connects the mouth to the stomach. Once in the stomach, food acids continue to breakdown the remaining partially digested food. The partially digested food then enters the small intestine where the liver and pancreas add their own digestive juices.

The pancreatic juices breakdown carbohydrates, proteins and fats while bile from the liver continues to breakdown the remaining fats, proteins and vitamins; these processes, combined with water, move the extracted mixture through the walls of the small intestine and into the blood stream.

If a child or adult has a negative reaction to foods with either sugar or *trans-fat*s, it could take the complete 72 hours for that reaction to subside.

Again, I mention, 'because of the lack of enzymes...' in the body to breakdown *trans*-fat, *trans-fat*s have nowhere to go; our bodies are simply not equipped to handle this fat. We know through scientific investigation that flat *trans*-fat molecules make their way into the human brain and other parts of the body such as the stomach. In their early years, if a child or children are living on a high *trans*-fat diet they may become very sick adults of the future.

## Following on with the scenario of Tom's brain, diagram 4, page 31

Tom is with his dad who has taken him to a fast food outlet where his dad wants to spend some quality time with his son. Let's assume the child is now eating a hash brown, some French fries and maybe a burger.

The artificial chemicals are starting to build in the child's system; Tom may start to feel different or start to misbehave.

### Trans-fats

11)

**Legend**
1) Healthy synapse
2) Dopamine
3) Adrenaline
4) Trans-fat molecule

Trans fat containing molecule may start to interfere with the synaptic sparks in the child's brain. This may lead to the hyperactivity and naughty behaviour exhibited by the child

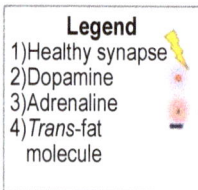

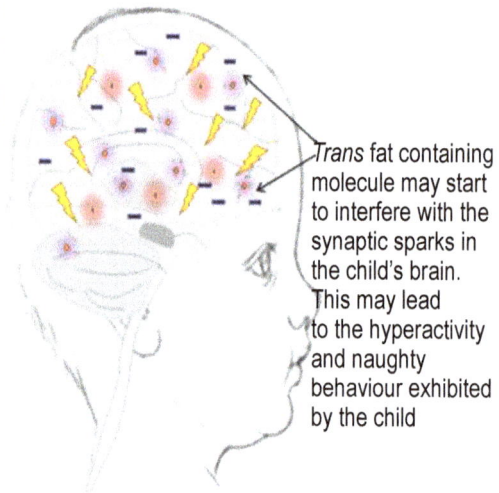

We can take this scenario further. In order to regain the child's attention, Tom is offered a fruit or milk drink. This will have a range of additives, some of which you will not be familiar with. An additive widely used in children's drinks is: 242 Dimethyl dicarbonate (DMDC). This is a synthetic additive and used as a yeast inhibitor; is poisonous and toxic and used in many beverages including children's juices. It also causes cancer.

**From the junk food, there's now an accumulation of different manufactured food chemicals working inside the child's head, their body, including their gut.**

**Food additives are now added to the treat**

12)

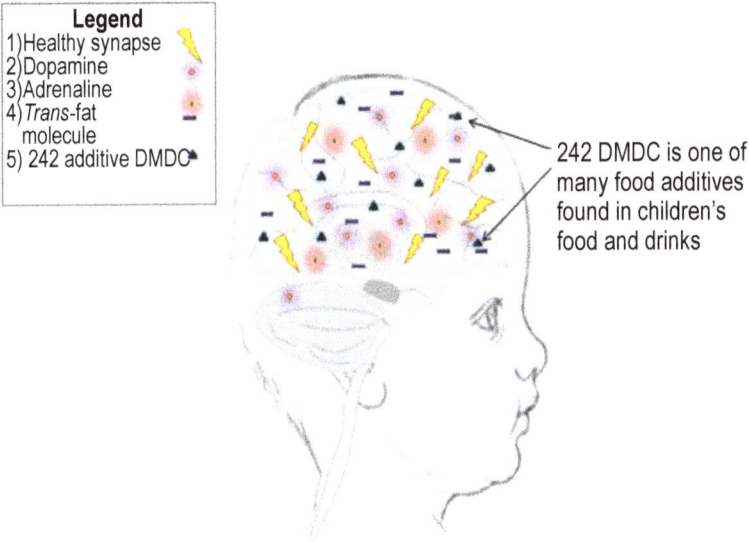

Legend
1) Healthy synapse
2) Dopamine
3) Adrenaline
4) *Trans*-fat molecule
5) 242 additive DMDC

242 DMDC is one of many food additives found in children's food and drinks

Like so many additives found in children's food and drinks, 242 (DMDC) is a synthetic product used by food manufacturers to produce the right appeal, selling colour, flavour and texture. Each mouthful swallowed may release more dopamine which may also lead to an adrenaline rush which the child experiences.

**Devils come in different colours and food packaging**

Often walking around the supermarket, I see a child putting on a tantrum because they want mum or dad to buy the latest packet of biscuits, chips, cakes or doughnuts they've seen in television advertising.

As I've previously mentioned, when tested for *trans-fat*, doughnuts weighed in at a hefty 50 percent of *trans-fat* content. They are colourful with iced toppings, coloured sprinkles, chocolate sprinkles and more decorative ideas.

Very few cakes are made without the ingredient of *trans-fat*s. Bakers and cake manufacturers like to use *trans-fat*s because they are cheap, and when baked, produce the finished product that stimulates *'mouth and eating appeal'*. The textures are tempting and have a golden glow. This can be seen in croissants, freshly baked rolls, brioche and other bread or cake products.

The visual sensation at seeing a cake in a cake shop allows you to salivate and even before buying the product, you can already taste it in your mouth. This is what effective marketing does.

You are not alone, millions of people around the world, including your children and family members go through the same processes when they see or spot a cake or a gastronomic delight, they particularly like to eat.

Now, please think, how your child thinks and feels when they see something sweet, fatty and want to eat it. If your child puts on a tantrum because they want to eat a sweet, gooey cake or any other mass market food product in the future, you will know your child has already developed a habit for this product. It's their brain demanding, once visually stimulated, from the 'pleasure centre', the food or drink they want.

Once the child has the taste, feels the texture in their mouth as they start to eat or drink, then start to swallow the product, they will possibly behave. You will know by these signs that you are indeed helping to create more bad habits for the child. Once satisfied, the child's brain will be quiet until the next time they see the stimulant; then they will start to crave to eat or drink the product again.

Once a routine is established, (this may be daily), it will be difficult to break.

Fast take away food chains are very familiar with creating this **'need or want'** in children and younger adults. They do it through extremely effective advertising and marketing.

### The brain of a child when it's been eating and drinking at a fast take away food outlet – the scenario, the reality

As Tom's meal continues and with extra swallowing of a sugary and an additive added drink, he will experience more dopamine demands and may exhibit other behaviours that are not a general characteristic of the child.

# An overloaded child's system

13)

**Legend**
1) Healthy synapse
2) Dopamine
3) Adrenaline
4) *Trans*-fat molecule
5) 242 additive DMDC
6) More dopamine
   is released

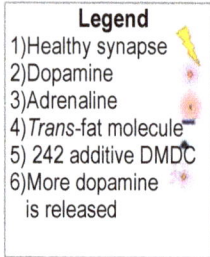

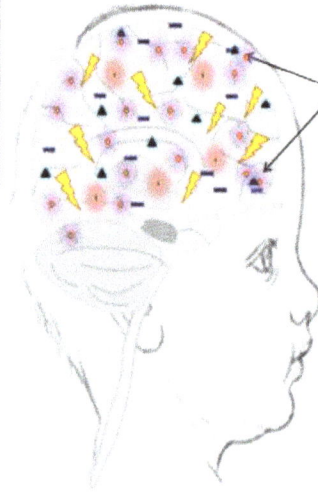

A demand signal is given and more dopamine is released with ingesting the sugary drink

For a short period of the time, the child will feel the pleasure of what they have ingested. Then, they may start to fidget and start to show nervousness in their behaviour. They start to play with the food in the wrapper and may occasionally eat a part of the hash brown or a chip. They become bored and are trying to cope with what is going on inside their head and body.

Without medically and invasive research, we have little evidence to measure when it comes to children eating junk food. Non-invasively, we can however, measure children's behaviours and the responses they have to foods eaten and drinks swallowed.

**Additives do their deed**

Foods can be labelled as natural when they do indeed have additives added. In the earlier part of the book I have mentioned: '*A food or drink manufacturer does not have to notify the consumer, if the additive is less than 5 percent'*.

**Giving you some idea of how additives work**

Additives – A product your child is eating may have the minimum additive of 4.99 percent. Let's look at the sums:

1. One Hash brown – 4.99 percent
2. A few French fries – 4.99 percent
3. A small burger – 4.99 percent
4. A fruit drink or milk shake – 4.99 percent
5. A biscuit or two – 4.99 percent.

If your child has a doughnut, you can be assured that the doughnut contents are at least 50 percent of *trans-fat*! Not good.

The few foods above, excluding the doughnut, already show the child has eaten four to five times the recommended volume of additives within one meal. Of course portion size, age and size of the child and other variables need to be considered but this information will allow you to rethink the food your child or children eat.

**Additives**

I have researched over 300 additives in bringing this book together. Some, I admit, have frightened me to death. Can it be possible, that food manufacturers are getting away with this? And 'Yes' they are.

## The poisoning truth – *trans-fats* combined with food additives

14)

**Legend**
1) Healthy synapse
2) Dopamine
3) Adrenaline
4) *Trans*-fat molecule
5) 242 additive DMDC
6) More dopamine is released
7) 102 Additive Tartrazine
8) 122 C114720
9) 150c Caramel
10) 514 Sodium sulphates

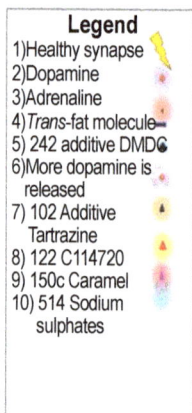

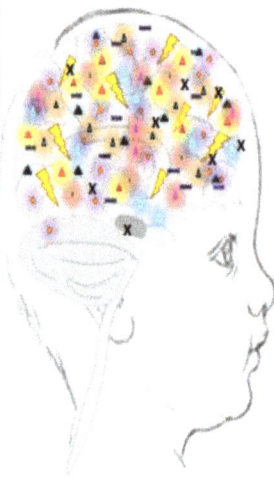

Some of the many additives found in children's processed food and drink:

102 Tartrazine
112 C114720
150c Caramel III
242 DMDC
514 Sodium sulphate

It takes a graphic description to shock us into action. Is it any wonder that some children have difficulty coping when the culmination of food additives, as seen in the above image, are working inside their systems? Because we can't see what additives are doing inside the head or body of our child or children, we make the assumption that all is well, when 'it is far from well'.

108

**Starting with the additive numbers seen in the diagram on page 108.**

Additive:

- **102 Tartrazine** – is a food colour derived from **coal tar**. Approved in New Zealand and Australia. To mention but a few products where this product is used in children's food:

  - Breakfast cereals
  - Crisps
  - Iced lollies
  - Macaroni cheese
  - Fizzy drinks
  - Pasta
  - Pancake mix and more. **Avoid**

Leads to hyperactivity, depression, learning difficulties and behavioural problems.

- **122 Azorubine or carmoisine, C114720** – is an artificial food colour derived from **coal tar**. Approved in New Zealand and Australia. To mention a few products additive 122 is used as an ingredient in children's food:

  - Sweets
  - Confectionary
  - Jellies
  - Marzipan. **Avoid**

Asthmatics should avoid. Leads to hyperactivity; is a carcinogen.

- **150c Caramel III** – can be made from genetically modified crops. Approved in New

Zealand and Australia. To mention a few products additive 150c is used as an ingredient in children's food:

- Cereals
- Confectionary, lollies and sweets
- Liquorice
- BBQ sauce
- Caramel flavourings. **Avoid**

In commercially and massed produced food products, caramel is made from **synthetic i**ngredients.

Will cause hyperactivity, is also linked to Attention Deficit Hyperactivity Disorder (ADHD). Is also linked to other illnesses.

- **242 Dimethyl dicarbonate DMDC** – is a synthetic and dangerous toxin and yeast exhibitor. On alert in New Zealand and Australia. To mention a few products additive 242 is used as an ingredient in children's drinks:

  - Fruit juices sold and marketed intentionally for child consumption
  - Carbonated drinks
  - Non-carbonated drinks
  - Flavoured waters. **Avoid**

Can cause irritation and swelling to the eyes and skin. Can also cause breathing difficulties; has been known to cause death if the fumes are inhaled.

For further information on drink additives found in children's drinks, please go to page 141.

- **514 Sodium sulphates, (i) Sodium sulphate, (ii) Sodium hydrogen sulphate or Sulphate of soda** – is commercially prepared from the salt of sulphuric acid. 514 is used as an ingredient in children's foods:

  - Sweets
  - Lollies
  - Biscuits
  - Confectionary
  - Chewing gum. **Avoid**

Is a dangerous additive for children who suffer with asthma and those who have breathing problems. May cause skin and eye irritation.

There are many more additives in children's food; just a few are mentioned here. Please go to Chapter Four, for a complete breakdown of additive information.

**The young offenders**

On page 11, I spoke about the young offenders I counselled and taught in the United Kingdom. Let us now take this a little further. The young offenders had problems in staying alert or completing any tasks on time. They had problems with concentration and little ability for the analysis of problems.

Given the young males' diet of deep-fried foods these problems are not surprising outcomes.

Studies have found that young males between the age of 20-45 years of age are the majority that eat at fast take away food outlets. Research also shows that their reaction time is a lot slower after eating a high *trans-fat* meal. Most fast food outlets sell their meals with a sugary soft drink or highly sweetened milk-based drink. All of which contain additives, fats and sugars and contribute to slow reaction time from the time of ingesting. If the poor eating habit continues, the outcome, as seen in the latest evidence of the seventeen-year-old male in the United Kingdom, now legally blind and deaf teenager with irreversible ill health.

## The devils gather

If you have grown up and, as a child, had fast take away meals as a regular part of your diet and are between the ages of 20 to 45 years, you may be in for a long journey to health recovery. I'm not only talking about young males but also females.

In her studies, Professor Golomb has referred to *'gaining weight, more aggression and heart disease.'*

If you've had relationship problems in your life, it would be wise to look at your diet. Equally so, if you are having problems with employment – you fly off the handle and get angry far beyond what is reasonable. In a fit of rage, you may even walk away from your current employment. These actions may relate to the food you are eating or drink you are swallowing.

Because our gut is inextricable linked to our brain all of the above behaviours may show themselves at the most inappropriate times.

We are, as working human beings, a combination of chemical reactions. For a healthy, satisfying life we need to keep our good chemicals in balance. When eating an anti-balance combination of chemicals, (food too, is a combination of chemicals), we upset the human system. Sugar and fat spoken of in these first two chapters are anti-balance chemicals; they need to be known about and guidelines need to be in place in the food supply chain so that people can protect themselves from eating the poison within the manufactured food goods sold.

Young males are high on the spectrum in the research carried out so far. Their demand and desire or cravings for fast, *trans-fat*, take away food is evident when travelling on highways and seeing the number of people, males in particular, in queues at roadside services.

The habit of eating *trans-fat*s is related to:

1. The taste buds in your mouth. Remember, we are programmed to like fat. When we were in evolution thousands if not millions of years ago, fat was in short supply. At that point we gained a taste for fat. Fat kept us warm in winter, the brain also felt good because it was the friendly and unprocessed *trans*-fat from wild animals and plants that made our bodies feel nourished and well.

2. From the taste buds to the stomach. Good fat is satisfying and gives us energy and helps to keep us healthy. *Your taste buds only exist in your mouth, not in your stomach!*

3. Your brain's 'pleasure centre' is in demand when unhealthy fat and sugar are consumed. (The brain does not discriminate between authentic and synthetic fat; it's the enzymes in the gut that appear to do the discrimination.) The brain's 'pleasure centre' when in demand

releases dopamine which creates more demands. Your brain does not register the good from bad chemistry of foods eaten. It's only when you become ill and you know you have health problems that you take action to rectify your health situation!

**Through life – a young person's reaction to *trans*-fat – as the child matures, habits are established – the scenario becomes a way of life**

15)

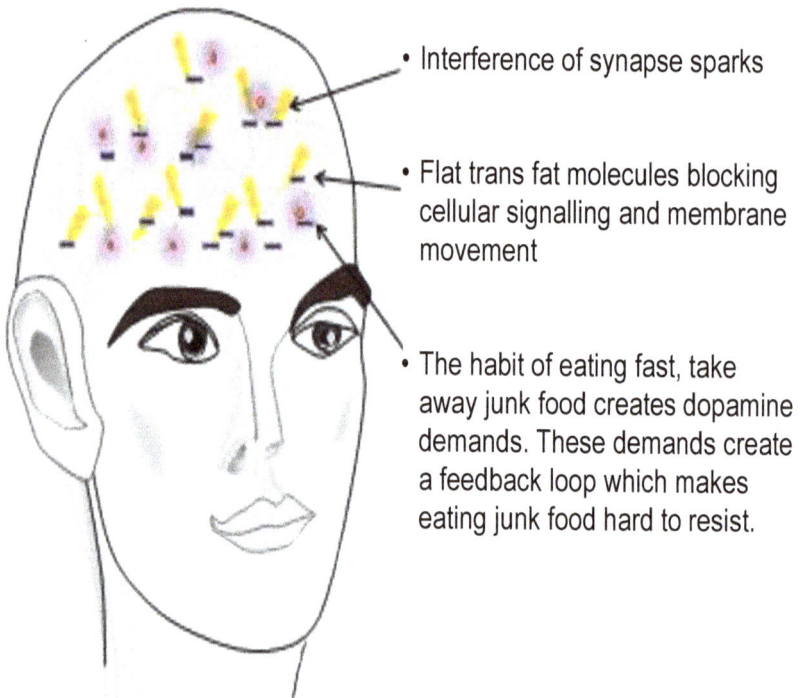

- Interference of synapse sparks

- Flat trans fat molecules blocking cellular signalling and membrane movement

- The habit of eating fast, take away junk food creates dopamine demands. These demands create a feedback loop which makes eating junk food hard to resist.

**_Trans-fat_ does nothing for your longevity**

Through eating excessive _trans_-fat, like other habits you develop, you become co-dependent on the feeling you receive from the 'pleasure centre' in your brain. _Trans-fat_s give you nothing apart from weight, more weight, ill health, the lack of fulfilling your future by dying prematurely.

**'Where are the advantages in this prospect you have to ask yourself?'**

**Age + trans-fats = poor health and ageing**

16)

• _Trans_ fat molecule numbers in your body system and brain increase

• Age accelerates and you look older than you are

• Your skin loses its elasticity and doesn't readily heal if cut

• Because of weight gain you have trouble exercising and walking

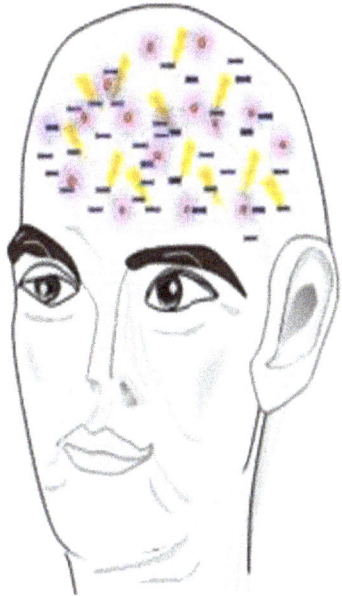

**Your physical inside body is older than your years**

Because of the *trans*-fat build up:

- Your heart goes into poor health
- You have a cholesterol build up in the arteries
- You have excess body fat on your stomach
- Fat starts to accumulate on your arms, legs, thighs and backside.

Other factors include:

- Poor memory and recall
- Poor reaction time
- Bad habits build on bad habits

**Your creation of bad habits are killing you**

You can reverse this problem – get rid of the *trans-fat*s in your diet.

When *trans-fat*s are nonexistent in your blood:

- You have a healthy blood flow
- You feel well
- You can run, exercise and
- Do the things that keep you happy.

You have the will to live and look forward to the challenge or next adventure.

**A healthy blood flow**

When your blood flow is clear your blood moves freely in and around your blood stream and you feel the difference.

**Healthy blood circulating around and through your body**

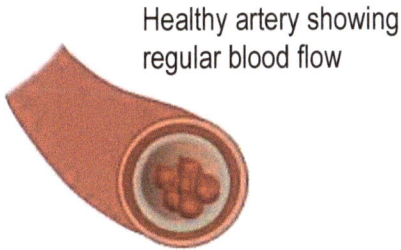

Healthy artery showing regular blood flow

As the blood flows it has the required oxygen to travel to your lungs, brain and other areas of your body.

Your body has developed to keep you well. It does all it can to maintain a healthy system, if you want to help to destroy this system, keep eating *trans*-fat!

**The devil in the *trans*-fat -** cholesterol build up in an artery

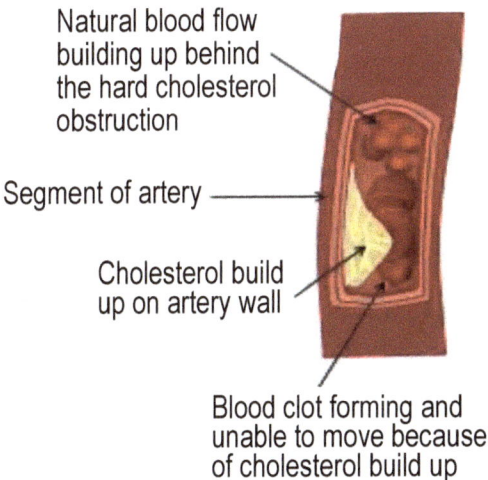

Natural blood flow building up behind the hard cholesterol obstruction

Segment of artery

Cholesterol build up on artery wall

Blood clot forming and unable to move because of cholesterol build up

**_Trans-fat_ is not body friendly, it is a devil**

By not being aware of what you are eating, you are contributing to your own poor health and to the wealth of the product manufacturers who sell a combination of _trans-fat_ products and label these products as food, when in fact they are selling poison to the greater community.

Many of the Western illnesses including: heart disease, Type 2 Diabetes, metabolic syndrome and arthritis can be attributed to the over processing of food, the manipulation of fats and increased sugar content.

A six-year study on monkeys given '_a high trans-fat diet caused insulin resistance, abnormal high belly fat to develop and elevated fructose levels._'[49] More research needs to be done in these areas. There are now clear warning signs that _trans-fat_s could do more harm than good.

**Your brain and the brains of our future generations**

With regard to junk and fast take away food, including those foods prepared using _trans-fat_s, there's a great deal of clinical research being done around the world. Evidence is pointing to the molecular changes in the food when natural food is processed, re-processed and changed to meet consumer demands. Consumer demands dictate the taste, quality, freshness and end selling price the manufacturers, supermarkets and fast food outlets work to. This combination of knowledge allows cheaper, fast food to be easily sold to the greater world population.

---

[49] https://www.ncbi.nlm.nih.gov/pubmed/17636085

Such molecular changes in food, can only lead to global illness and premature deaths. Our brains need healthy molecules with room to move; movement allows for cellular signalling and membrane movement allowing neurotransmitters to do their job. Flat *trans-fat*s restrict or hinder neurotransmitter information, therefore, a human response is seen as slow or a reaction does not take place. All of which will contribute to a poorer, weaker world population.

## Our planet

Tree logging corporations are stripping out land, including large forests, to grow more plants such as palm for the production of cheap palm oil. Food corporations are using hydrogenation or partial hydrogenation, including palm oil, to create *trans*-fat oils. This manipulation of a product has a two-fold effect:

- The clearance of forests and farmland to grow cheap palm for an insatiable junk food worldwide market place making the populations of the world sick.

- The destruction of animal habitat of that country which leads to the eradication of already threatened or endangered animal species.

## No requirement on *trans*-fat labelling in Australia

In 2011 a Federal Government review recommended labelling or a total phase out of *trans-fat*s by 2013. We are now in 2019/20 and consumers are still left in the dark with regards to the *trans-fat* content in the foods they buy and eat.

*'In Australia, there is no requirement for manufacturers to list trans-fats as an ingredient on packaging because it falls under the category of unsaturated fats.'* [50] said Dr Rosemary Stanton, Nutritionist.

As you now know, a *trans*-fat is a saturated fat that causes ill health and death and the reason being: the hydrogen carbon has been re-programmed by partial or full hydrogenation to meet a manufacturer's requirements to make cheap food.

*'For a 2,000 calorie per day diet, the trans-fat limit is 2 grams daily.'*[51] With just a spread of margarine on your daily sandwich you can soon overload you body with this fat. You may add to your food intake: a bought biscuit or cake for morning tea, have a pie, croissant or brioche for lunch. On the way home, you call in and buy some hot chips or a burger. All of these foods contain *trans-fat*s as part of their regular ingredients.

If your diet resembles some of what has been spoken of in the previous pages, your recommended 2 grams of *trans-fat* a day has been increased by up to 30 times of the recommended fat intake. To give you some idea of how this works we need to look at how much margarine is contained in a regular tub.

Normally, people buy a 250gm tub, so let us do the math. Please see the following page.

---

[50] https://thenewdaily.com.au. 19/05/2018.
[51] Dr. Tina M. St. John, Updated December 07, 2018. https://healthyeating.sfgate.com

**Margarine – possibly the biggest *trans*-fat devil in the modern diet**

**Your 2 grams of *trans-fat* a day**

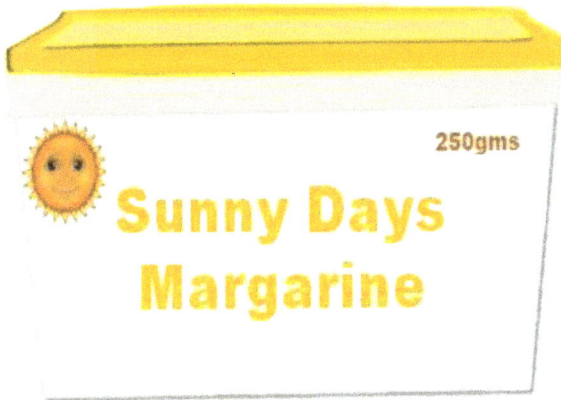

Fictitious brand name

A tub of commercially manufactured margarine holds 250 grams.

Your recommended daily allowance is 2 grams of *trans-fat* per day this would represent 14 grams eaten over a week. If you were to eat half the container of margarine over seven days, you would eat 125 grams. You are consuming approximately nine times more than the recommended weekly allowance.

Along with other *trans-fat*s you consume your intake of fat would be dangerously high. If you do this on a regular basis you are inviting heart disease, obesity and other illnesses, including Diabetes Type 2 into your life.

## Doughnuts – a devil and a killer

Doughnuts have added *trans*-fat to their dough and then cooked in *trans*-fat oil. Studies have revealed doughnuts can increase their *trans*-fat content by up to 50 percent or more.

## Moving forward

The United States and five member countries of the European Union now have a virtual ban on *trans-fat*s or have reduced the recommended *trans*-fat to 2 grams a day across all manufactured food products. These countries include: Denmark, Austria, Hungary, Iceland, Norway and Switzerland. Denmark has seen several health benefits by practically banning *trans-fat*s altogether:

- *'Trans-fat intake decreased among all age groups and is now one tenth of the level when the ban was adopted.'*
- *Within one year, most products on the Danish market were able to comply with the new limit of 2 grams of trans-fat per* **one hundred grams of fat***.*
- *The overall nutritional profile of food products could improve, including the increases in use of healthier fats (such as monounsaturated or polyunsaturated fats), according to the Danish Ministry of Food, Agriculture and Fisheries.*
- *The drop in trans-fat consumption may partly account for the significant decrease in mortality from cardiovascular diseases recently experienced in Denmark.* [52]

---

[52] http://www.euro.who.int/en/media-centre

For further information, contact: Tina Kiaer, Communications Officer, WHO, Regional Office for Europe.

## Australia

To repeat: *'In Australia, there is no requirement for manufacturers to list trans-fats as an ingredient on packaging because it falls under the category of unsaturated fats.'* said, Dr Rosemary Stanton, Nutritionist. https://thenewdaily.com.au. 19/05/2018.

With the evidence presented in this one book alone, a revision of *trans-fat* recommendations needs to immediately take place in Australia, New Zealand and other countries.

## Foods with *trans*-fat as an ingredient or foods cooked in *trans-fat*

Manmade *trans*-fats have a different chemical formation in hydrogen atoms. It is this difference that causes:

- Obesity
- Sickness
- Cholesterol related illnesses
- Diabetes and
- Detrimental effects on blood vessels.

## Children eating *trans*-fat – the unseen devil

Added to the above, think about the food you and your family daily eat. If you have children, look at the food they take to school in their lunch packs. Do they have sugary drinks that give you the impression they have no added sugar? Read the label. Does the packet of chips in their lunch include the word: *trans-fat* content? Possibly not because the chips fall under the minimum amount of *trans-fat* content and do not require the manufacturer to give you the information on their labelling facts. As has been seen on the previous page, *trans-fats* in Australia fall under the category of unsaturated fats which does nothing to help the Australian consumer or population.

### A healthy child with a healthy brain loves to learn, play and have fun.

**So far, let's look at the accumulation of sugar, *trans-fat* and additives in Tom's brain and body system as he eats a take-away meal.**

Remembering there can be 100 million molecules to an inch; the diagrams below are distinguishing the chemistry taking place once sugar, *trans-fats* and some additives are consumed.

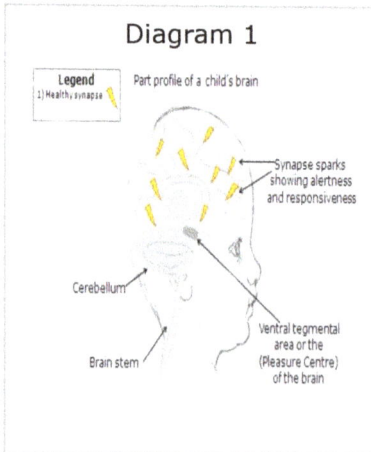

Diagram 1

Legend
1) Healthy synapse

Part profile of a child's brain

Synapse sparks showing alertness and responsiveness

Cerebellum

Brain stem

Ventral tegmental area or the (Pleasure Centre) of the brain

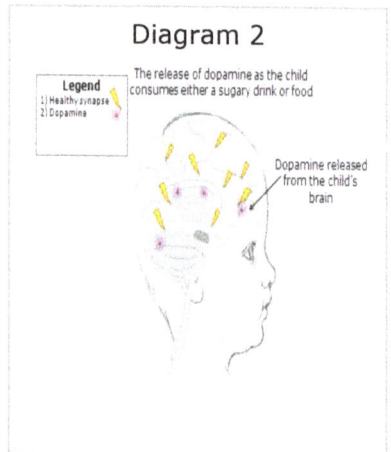

Diagram 2

Legend
1) Healthy synapse
2) Dopamine

The release of dopamine as the child consumes either a sugary drink or food

Dopamine released from the child's brain

Diagram 3

Legend
1) Healthy synapse
2) Dopamine

Sugary substances

As sugary substances leach into the child's system, more dopamine is released from the child's brain

Diagram 4

Legend
1) Healthy synapse
2) Dopamine
3) Adrenaline

The release of adrenaline

Adrenaline is released which makes the child hyperactive

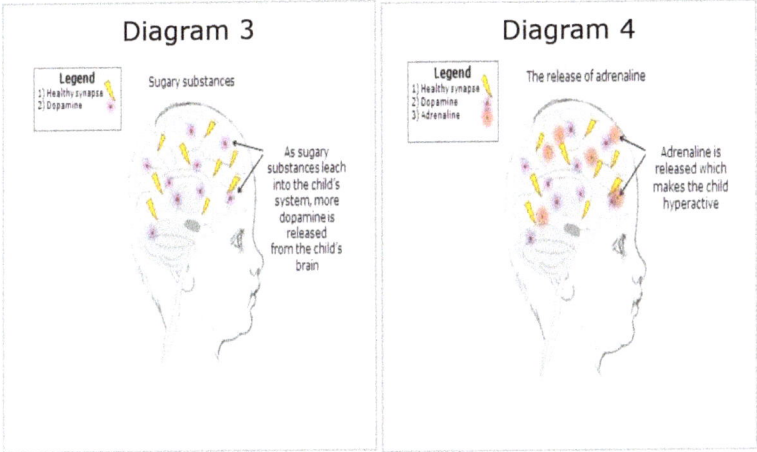

Technology is still limited in the research that can be done with regard to the human brain. The brain diagrams within this book have been designed to raise awareness to the reaction that may take place when sugar, *trans-fats*, additives and other poisons are ingested into the human system.

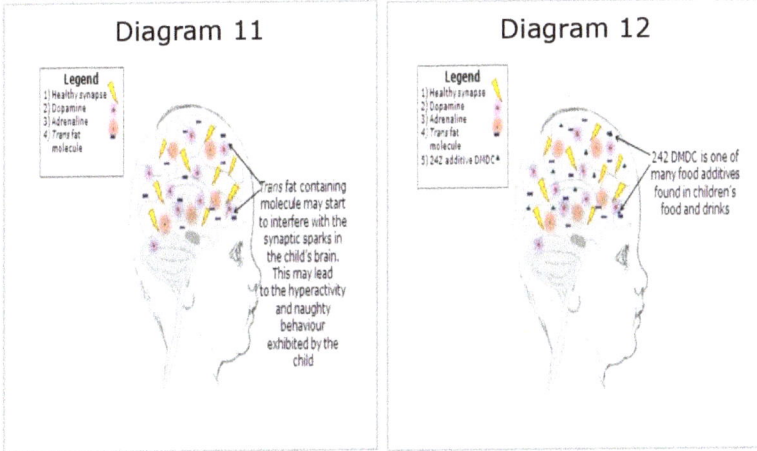

Diagram 11

Legend
1) Healthy synapse
2) Dopamine
3) Adrenaline
4) Trans fat molecule

Trans fat containing molecule may start to interfere with the synaptic sparks in the child's brain. This may lead to the hyperactivity and naughty behaviour exhibited by the child

Diagram 12

Legend
1) Healthy synapse
2) Dopamine
3) Adrenaline
4) Trans fat molecule
5) 242 additive DMDC*

242 DMDC is one of many food additives found in children's food and drinks

### Diagram 13

**Legend**
1) Healthy synapse
2) Dopamine
3) Adrenaline
4) Trans fat molecule
5) 242 additive DHDC
6) More dopamine is released

A demand signal is given and more dopamine is released with ingesting the sugary drink

### Diagram 14

**Legend**
1) Healthy synapse
2) Dopamine
3) Adrenaline
4) Trans fat molecule
5) 242 additive DHDC
6) More dopamine is released
7) 102 Additive Tartrazine
8) 122 C114720
9) 150c Caramel
10) 514 Sodium sulphates

Some of the many additives found in children's processed food and drink:

102 Tartrazine
122 C114720
150c Caramel III
514 Sodium sulphate

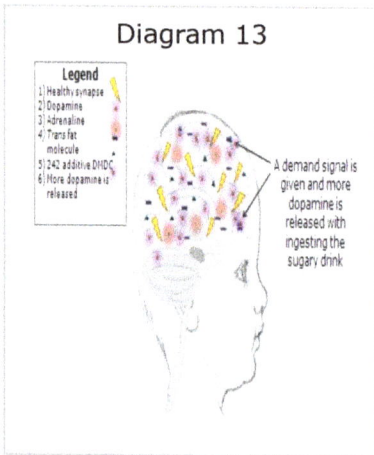

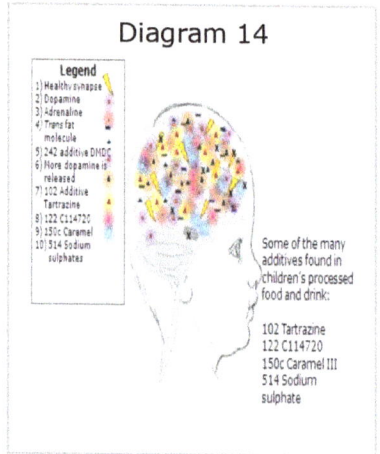

As can be seen in the last two chapters, the accumulation of poisons within our food affect both children and adults, the only solution is to limit their intake.

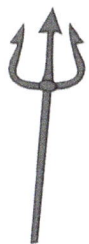

# The

# Bliss

# Point

## The 'Bliss Point' fats

Like all foods that appeal to our taste buds there has to be a 'bliss point' appeal built into the marketing of the product.' *Trans-fats* help to create the visual appeal that makes you want to buy and eat.

## Visual impact:

- Freshness: does it look good enough to eat and is the colour of the product appealing?
- Texture: does the crust look golden brown like freshly baked bread?
- If a meat pie: does the gravy look dark and rich or is light and insipid?
- If a frozen fruit pie in a supermarket refrigerator: does it look like the word description? You won't know until you get it home and remove the pie from the packaging.

## The visual sensations as you imagine eating the food:

- The colour and texture of the food
- Imagining the crunchiness of the pastry or sensation as it enters your mouth. You may have a prior experience and want to re-live that experience.
- Feeling the satisfaction of the food after its eaten

## The 'bliss point' reaching its goal

The 'bliss point' can only reach its goal if it has the required amounts of salt, fat and sugar in the product to make it desirable to the consumer to eat. A few products that focus on the 'Bliss Point' would be bakeries in their production of:

- Brioche
- Croissants
- Breads
- Pies
- Cakes and
- Biscuits

Fast food outlets create regular changing marketing images of their food with each image giving you the messages:

- 'This is good for you'
- 'This is healthy for you' despite it having been cooked in *trans-fat*
- 'You'll be one of the crowd if you eat this.' (I've mentioned the advertisement on page 99, seen over Christmas 2018).

Marketing for junk food always include the images of:

- golden looking deep-fried fish or chicken
- golden cooked edges on wood fired pizzas
- crunchy and golden cooked chips or deep fries
- golden coloured, under the soft icing, of deep-fried doughnuts
- golden coloured biscuits and cakes and more tempting images.

## Marketing – enhancing the 'Bliss Point'

When a food product is being developed by food manufacturers, the 'bliss point' has all of the previously mentioned trigger points to your emotions built into its marketing and development. Prior to my research and writing this book, on many occasions I've taken a frozen fruit pie out of its box only to be disappointed by the image I'm looking at. The image did not represent the image portrayed on the packaging.

If the 'bliss point' fails in any way, the consumer will be very reluctant to buy that product a second time and consumerism is what large food corporations rely on to sell their products. Repeat customers are the only way they can financially survive.

# The devil's persuasion

## The devil of *trans-fats*

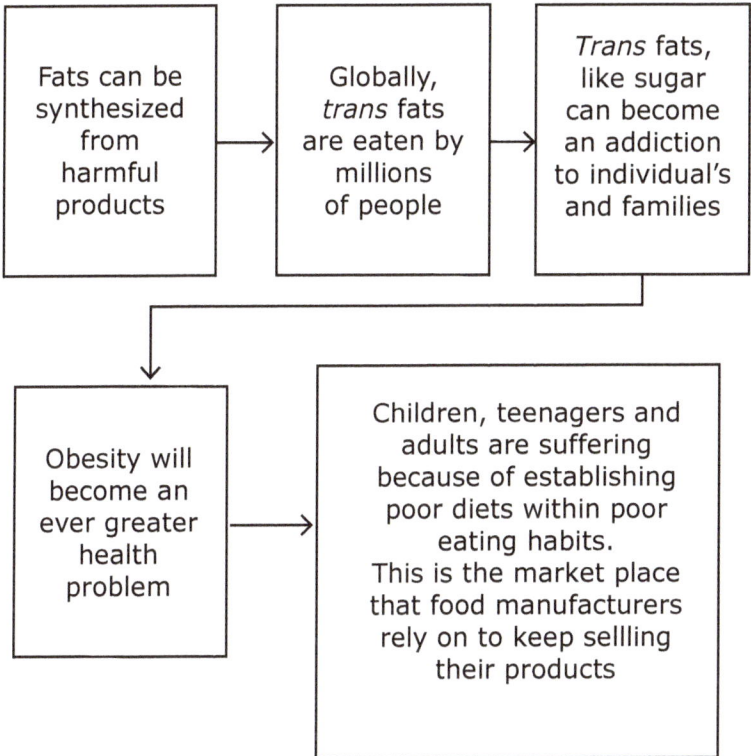

```
┌──────────────────┐     ┌──────────────────┐     ┌──────────────────┐
│  Fats can be     │     │   Globally,      │     │  Trans fats,     │
│  synthesized     │     │   trans fats     │     │  like sugar      │
│  from         ───┼──→  │   are eaten by───┼──→  │  can become      │
│  harmful         │     │   millions       │     │  an addiction    │
│  products        │     │   of people      │     │  to individual's │
│                  │     │                  │     │  and families    │
└──────────────────┘     └──────────────────┘     └──────────────────┘

        ┌──────────────────┐     ┌──────────────────────────────────┐
        │  Obesity will    │     │  Children, teenagers and         │
        │  become an       │     │  adults are suffering            │
        │  ever greater ───┼──→  │  because of establishing         │
        │  health          │     │  poor diets within poor          │
        │  problem         │     │  eating habits.                  │
        │                  │     │  This is the market place        │
        └──────────────────┘     │  that food manufacturers         │
                                 │  rely on to keep sellling        │
                                 │  their products                  │
                                 └──────────────────────────────────┘
```

**Your Notes**

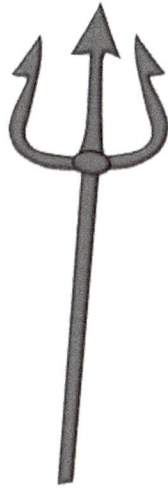

# Devils in
# Our Food

# Chapter Three ~

## The devils of table salt, caffeine and rice

**Salt**

Every cell in the human body needs to receive a small amount of natural salt from the food that's eaten. Our body relies on natural salt to help maintain blood circulation, equalize bone density and maintain blood sugar levels.

**Fast running table salt**

On the supermarket shelves there are many salt products available. I'm going to concentrate on fast, running, table salt used in the restaurant industry, in fast food chain outlets and the manufacture of their products. Table salt is also used in the mass production of commercially manufactured food including:

- Snacks
- Chips of many flavours
- Corn chips
- Health bars
- Some ice creams
- Confectionary
- Children's drinks
- Fizzy drinks
- Breads, rolls and dough products manufactured in the bakery industry and
- Cake mixes

Pre-cooked foods including:

- Baked potato products
- Pre-cooked meals
- Desserts
- Pies and
- Cakes

Table salt is also used in:

- School, college and university canteens and dining halls
- Residential homes, hospitals and hotels, food catering outlets
- Catering for air, train and coach travel
- Roadside services
- Public events where catering is part of the venue and other venues where food is served.

Most, if not all, manufactured and processed food would contain fast running **table salt**.

## Table salt is a devil

Apart from naturally occurring rock or sea salt, smooth running refined table salt is used in many family homes. The majority of table salt is a synthetic product that is made from **crude oil flakes** which are the residue of oil diggings. For refinement, the flakes are heated to 1,200 degrees Fahrenheit.

Other manufactured table salt may include mineral halite or rock salt. Processing methods are a key concern to their health validity.

Free running table salt looks like salt, tastes like salt but is not salt. It is purely an imitation of natural salt which is used in food, beverage, and confectionary manufacture.

Common table salt, though tasting similar to rock and sea salt, is completely artificial and offers none of the benefits that naturally occurring rock or sundried sea salt offer. Through the lack of heating sea salt maintains its natural minerals and beneficial properties.

To maintain its free-flowing ability, synthetic table salt has anti-caking agents added during the manufacturing process. Also added:

- Synthetic iodine
- Monosodium glutamate (MSG), sodium aluminate[53] (For further information breakdown on additives in salt please see Chapter Four: 330 Citric acid, 620 L-glutamic acid and 621 monsodium glutamate)
- Sodium bicarbonate
- Synthetic iodide
- Fluoride
- Potassium iodide
- Cyanide
- By-products of aluminium and
- Bleach

Bleach is used to whiten salt crystals and to influence the user, that what they are eating is a pure product. It is far from pure.

---

[53] In industry and in technical applications, sodium aluminate is used as an inorganic chemical. It is used as an effective source for aluminium hydroxide.

*'Table salt is a manufactured form of sodium called sodium chloride. Table salt is particularly hard on both the circulatory system and nervous system. It also wreaks havoc on the delicate balance of the lymph system in the body.'*[54]

The ill-health conditions associated with table salt are numerous, but to mention a few:

- Over time, will affect the lymph gland system
- Will affect the circulatory systems
- Raises blood pressure (hypertension)
- Allows the body to retain excess water
- Contributes to Diabetes Type 2
- Can create systematic imbalances causing gout and obesity
- Has dependency characteristics – you can become dependent on table salt – a synthetic and artificial product.

Like other synthetic additives, 'our guts do not have the enzymes...' to process refined table salt. Once eaten, your body has no way of discharging this poison from your system; it is possibly with you for life.

Other ill health outcomes include:

- Nervous disorders
- Apprehension
- Depression
- Kidney disorders
- Thyroid problems
- Heart problems or disease
- Muscle cramps and

---

[54] Dr Edward Group - https://www.globalhealingcenter.com

- Goitre conditions

## Natural caffeine

Most people look forward to their daily cup of coffee. Natural caffeine can help in the movement of bowel movements and help to keep you regular.

Caffeine (natural or synthetic) is also added to tea, energy drinks, many soft drinks, chocolate and confectionary and possibly other foods and drinks!

## 9 Side effects of too much caffeine

1) `Anxiety

2) Insomnia

3) Digestive disorders

4) Muscle breakdown

5) Addiction

6) High blood pressure

7) Rapid heart rate

8) Fatigue and

9) Frequent urination and urgency. [55]

---

[55] Written by Franziska Spritzler, RD CDE 14/08/2017. https://www.healthline.com

## Synthetic caffeine – a devil

The global demand for caffeine is high and expensive, synthetic caffeine can be and is used to replace the natural product.

Synthetic caffeine was first produced in 1942 during WWII by the Nazis in Germany. Synthetic caffeine is cheap to produce and can be manufactured by unregistered producers. To produce synthetic caffeine, ammonia[56] is converted into urea this undergoes many steps of change including exposure to methylene chloride, ethyl acetate and carbon dioxide. When the original processing is completed the substance glows. The glow is removed by rinsing with acetic acid, chloroform, sodium carbonate and sodium nitrite. These processes produce synthetic caffeine found in many foods and drinks available on the supermarket shelf, in road side services, cafes, general food outlets including airports, train and coach stations, fast food take away outlets and many other retail food and convenience food stores.

Synthetic caffeine is used in many health drinks and health supplement foods. It's also used in a wide range of soft drinks sold in the worldwide marketplace.

All synthetic caffeine is made in China with little to no regulation on the materials used in the manufacture of the product. Without regulation, mistakes will happen.

In Australia and New Zealand, food and drink manufacturers have no legal requirement to state that synthetic caffeine is used in their product. By looking

---

[56] Ammonia is a colourless gas – can be manufactured or naturally produced.

at the product label you will see the word caffeine – what type of caffeine will not be stated.

Many parents and teachers don't necessarily know about the young teenage adults that drink synthetic caffeine in manufactured drinks on the way to school. Of course, there is more to a synthetic caffeinated drink than just caffeine there are also the other additives to consider.

**The flying bottle**

I had a very disruptive senior student in one of my classes. He was agitated coming into the classroom and most students seemed to avoid him. He carried his largish bottle of caffeine loaded drink in his hand and promptly put it on the desk, where he sat at the back of the room. Despite my requests, *'Please put that bottle into your bag or on the floor.'* The bottle of drink remained firmly on the desk and in my sight.

After a short time, and as we worked through the objectives of the lesson, he started to annoy the students close to him. He then became ever more disruptive. The Assistant Principal was asked to come to the room and remove the boy. This happened; the boy returned to my lesson a little time later.

This type of behaviour disrupts a good lesson and the students who want to learn are denied their right to education because of the acts of one student – very unfair.

Hoping to continue with the lesson on the boy's return, the disruptive behaviour continued. Most of the students were trying to do their class work through the disruptions. I went and spoke quietly to him and thought he would settle down. As I returned to my desk, the bottle sitting on his desk was thrown through the air narrowly missing my head.

The Assistant Principal and Principal came to the classroom to remove the boy; he was later expelled from the school.

We don't know what goes on in some young people's lives. They may be carrying many forms of hurt, anger, anguish and stress. The manufacturers of additive, sugar-loaded drinks are doing nothing to help the situation. Like alcohol, energy drinks and caffeinated drinks should have an age restriction clearly seen on the label.

The fact that teenagers can buy these drinks, over the counter, on the way to school should be banned.

## Additive devils in soft drinks and children's drinks

The list below identifies some of the additives added to manufactured and processed drinks. When synthetic caffeine is added, such combinations can create a lethal cocktail:

- **150a**   Caramel 1. Found in many soft drinks
- **150d**   Caramel IV. Found in soft and fizzy drinks
- **216**   Sodiupropyl p- hydroxybenzonate. Found in fruit cordials and juices
- **218**   Methylparaben or Methyl- p-hydroxybenzoate. Found in soft drinks and pineapple juice
- **220**   Sulphur dioxide. Found in juices and cordials

- **222**    Sodium bisulphite. Found in fruit and vegetable juices
- **223**    Sodium metabisulphate. Found in concentrate fruit and vegetable juices
- **224**    Potassium metabisulphite. Found fruit juices
- **225**    Potassium sulphite. Found in juices and cordials
- **242**    Dimethyl dicarbonate (DMDC). Found in children's juices, carbonated and non-carbonated drinks and flavoured water
- **243**    Ethyl lauroyl arginate. Found in fruit juices and other drinks
- **290**    Calcium sorbate. Found in fizzy and soft drinks
- **297**    Fumaric acid. Found in soft drinks
- **315**    Erythorbic acid. Found in dairy-based drinks
- **320**    Butylated hydroxyanisole (BHA). Found in soft drinks
- **328**    Ammonium lactate. Found in soft drinks
- **333**    Calcium citrate. Found in carbonated drinks
- **335**    Sodium tartrate. Found in carbonated drinks
- **336**    Potassium tartrates. Found in carbonated drinks
- **337**    Potassium sodium. Found in cola drinks
- **338**    Phosphoric acid. Found in cola like drinks and soda fizzy drinks
- **339**    Sodium phosphates. Found in cola drinks
- **350**    Sodium hydrogen malate. Found in all fruit drinks and soft drinks
- **351**    Potassium malates. Found in fruit drinks, soft drinks and fruit squash

- **352** Calcium malate. Found in fruit drinks and fruit squash
- **357** Potassium adipate. Found in all fruit drinks
- **410** Locust bean gum or carob bean gum. Found in soft drinks
- **414** Acacia or gum Arabic. Found in fruit drinks and squash
- **420** Sorbitol or sorbitol syrup. Found in low-calorie drinks
- **433** Polysorbate 80. Found in soft drinks
- **436** Polysorbate 65. Found in soft drinks
- **444** Sucrose acetate isobutyrate. Found in cloudy and flavoured drinks
- **445** Glycerol esters of rosin. Found in orange, fizzy canned drinks
- **463** Hydroxypropyl cellulose. Found in dairy drinks
- **446** Sodium carboxymethyl cellulose. Found in soft drinks
- **471** Mono- and di-glycerides of fatty acids. Found in hot chocolate mixes and drinks
- **500** Sodium bicarbonate. Found in soft and fizzy drinks
- **518** Magnesium sulphate. Found in many drinks
- **900a** Polydimethylsiloxane or dimethylpolysiloxane (PDMS). Found in milk shakes, smoothies, soft drinks and cordials
- **951** Aspartame, Nutrasweet, Equal. Found in powdered soft drinks
- **952** Cyclamates. Found in soft, fizzy fruit and diet drinks
- **954** Saccharins. Used in many drinks
- **956** Alitame. Found in water-based drinks and dairy-based drinks

- **961**    Neotame. Found in carbonated soft drinks
- **1413**    Phosphated distarch phosphate. Found in cola and soft drinks
- **1522**    Calcium lignosulphonate (40-65). Found, as a carrier in fruit-based drinks.

**(Please see Chapter Four, Page 154 for further information on additive numbers and their related information).**

### Rice and arsenic

It's difficult to believe that rice could come under any devil headings but it does. This food has been eaten for thousands of years, so why can rice be harmful to the human body?

Rice naturally thrives on the intake of arsenic which is a natural chemical element of many soils. We have thought for many years that *'rice is good for you'*. It appears now not to be the case.

Rice is added to many foods, including babies and children's, these include:

- Baby and toddler formulas
- Baby and toddler manufactured meals
- Baby and toddler manufactured desserts
- Cereal bars
- Energy bars
- Rice cakes for children and adults
- Rice syrup
- Rice flour
- Rice milk (which is often fortified with many vitamins and mineral additives)
- Rice breakfast cereals

- Rice-based cereals
- Rice-based convenient foods
- Rice bran oil
- Rice-based noodles
- Rice-based bread
- Rice-based pasta
- Rice vinegar and
- Rice-based alcoholic beverages

Brown rice appears to have the highest content of arsenic because of different growing locations and different growing methods.

Brian Jackson, analytical chemist,[57] led a study into the effects of arsenic in rice. Published in Environmental Health Perspectives, *'For people who occasionally eat a cereal bar, I don't see a problem.'* He continues, *'But for toddler formula, until we know what a safe arsenic level is, I recommend discontinuing that formula.'*[58] With no government guide lines in place as to the safe measurements of the toxicity of arsenic in food and the outcome from this poison, we must assume that eating rice is a health hazard.

Feeding babies on formula, toddlers and young children on rice crackers, rice-based foods or giving them rice-based milk is not an option until more research is forthcoming.
Babies, toddlers and children are more at risk from dangerous chemicals; they have smaller bodily systems to process the poison and are still physically developing. Until the age of five, their brains are still growing and establishing. At this point, we have no substantial studies that can verify the positive or

---

[57] Dartmouth Toxic Metals Superfund Research Program.
[58] The Salt https://www.npr.org

negative outcomes for a child when consuming food products containing arsenic. We don't know, at this point, what the long-term outcome for people consuming any form of poison or additive will be.

Further studies reveal daily eating half a cup of cooked rice is the same as drinking a litre of arsenic contaminated water.

Andrew Meharg, professor of biochemistry at the University of Aberdeen has been studying the people of Southeast Asia who have a daily consumption of rice. Meharg, found that arsenic polluted water wells are used to irrigate rice paddies *'the amount of arsenic in rice has increased tenfold in some areas of Bangladesh.'*[59]

Arsenic has been found in:

- Grape juice
- Apple juice and some
- Fruit juices

Arsenic naturally occurs in soils and on the earth's crust, however, arsenic can become a part of the growing process through:

1) Polluted waterways
2) Mining and industry discharge of waste and through
3) Agricultural chemicals, including pesticides used in farming and growing produce.

---

[59] The Salt https://www.npr.org

Until rice is farmed in a healthy, sustainable way, eating rice could pose many health problems and health hazards for the future.

It has been suggested, if eating rice, to soak overnight or for 24 hours, drain, cook and rinse well after cooking.

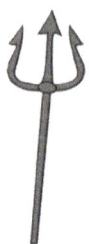

# The
# Bliss
# Point

## The 'Bliss Point' salt, caffeine and rice

All three products can contribute to our 'Bliss Point' as we eat and enjoy our food.

### Table salt

To maintain its healthy functions, each cell in the human body requires a fraction of salt. There is a natural demand from our body to have this product in our food. Our taste buds cannot tell the difference from synthetic or natural salt. It's not until the synthetic salt hits our gut that the true origins of the salt begin to unravel. This is possibly shown years later when our health starts to deteriorate, and we become sick.

Table salt is addictive and if the addiction is not restricted, the demand for table salt will increase.

### Caffeine and synthetic caffeine

Natural caffeine can be good for us but too much caffeine can have detrimental health outcomes. The nine side effects of caffeine have been spoken of earlier in this chapter. I've also spoken about synthetic caffeine. My research reveals facts not known by the general public. When buying your next soft drink either for yourself or for a member of your family, will you consider the caffeine in the drink and ask yourself: is it either synthetic or natural? Will you also see if the drink contains any other additives?

### Rice

Rice contains differing quantities of arsenic and to this day, there is no reliable data that says a certain quantity is healthy. As discussed, and until further research into the grain on its arsenic levels, it's suggested that babies and young children should not be given any form of rice food.

## The 'Bliss Point'

All three: table salt, caffeine (including synthetic caffeine), and rice work on the 'pleasure centres' of our brains'. Simply, because caffeine and salt are additives and in (the majority of cases, synthetic), they have a drug capability. Rice, on the other hand, when eaten, makes us feel comfortable. It is indeed a 'comfort food'. Just add some table salt to your rice dish, wash it down with a synthetic caffeine drink and you will possibly feel content and satisfied – you have now reached the 'Bliss Point' the food and beverage manufactures were aiming for.

It's when the demands from your brain's 'pleasure centre' go past the reality point, and over time, that problems in health and wellbeing come into your life.

## The devil's persuasion

### The devils in salt, caffeine and rice

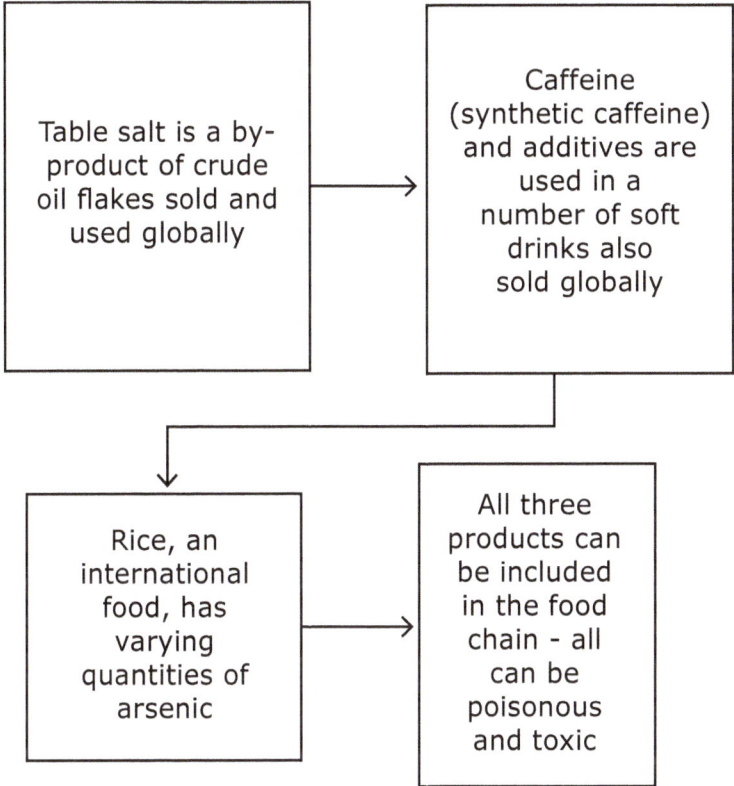

Table salt is a by-product of crude oil flakes sold and used globally

Caffeine (synthetic caffeine) and additives are used in a number of soft drinks also sold globally

Rice, an international food, has varying quantities of arsenic

All three products can be included in the food chain - all can be poisonous and toxic

## Your Notes

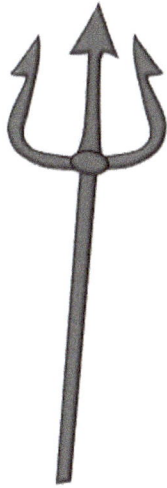

# Devils in
# Our Food

# Chapter Four ~
## *The devils of food additives*

### Understanding Additive E Numbers – Europe

E numbers are codes for substances that are permitted to be used as food additives for use within the European Union and the European Free Trade Association (EFTA). The 'E' stands for 'Europe'. Commonly found on food labels, their safety assessment and approval are the responsibility of the European Food Safety Authority (EFSA). Having a single unified list for food additives was first agreed upon in 1962 for food colouring. In 1964, the directives for preservatives were added, 1970 for antioxidants and 1974 for emulsifiers, stabilisers, thickeners and gelling agents.

### Understanding Additive Numbers – New Zealand and Australia

E numbers in New Zealand and Australia still have the same number representing the additive but the 'E' has been removed from the number. The number still corresponds with the European number codes.

Additives are made from different products some are synthesized, and some are manufactured through different extraction methods. Additives in the food we eat are:

- Colours
- Preservatives
- Antioxidants

154

- Artificial Sweeteners and
- Flavour Essences

*'Food additives are substances added intentionally to food stuffs to perform certain technological functions, for example to colour, to sweeten or to help preserve foods.'*[60]

Many foods have flavour enhancers, colour enhancers and other additives to appeal to our senses of: sight, smell, touch and taste. Smell happens in the olfactory bulb behind the nose. Your nose is highly sensitive to the smell of food, pheromones and hazards. If your 'pleasure centre' has been previously stimulated by something you've eaten and enjoyed, your desire to have that same taste again is heightened.

Your sense of smell will tell you when something doesn't taste right or if the taste is not compatible with what you like to eat or drink.

Manufacturers of food products know about the olfactory bulb and how to create the 'want' 'desire' and 'must have' when they are in research and development of food products. Many children's foods are decorative in many different colours and manufactures use many different strategies to make them appealing. They are also aware that the child is not the customer, the parents are the customers but to gain access to the parent and their money, they must gain access through the desires of the child. This is selling psychology.

---

[60] https://www.efsa.europa.eu

At the start and at intervals throughout the book I've mentioned my educator role. To expand on this topic, when in the classroom and when I look into the young faces of eight, nine, ten, and eleven-year old's I stop and think of their journey in life.

From my own experiences and remembering that age, life and the journey into adulthood puts many demands on a young person. Puberty is a demand of nature, a young person cannot avoid that journey, nor can they avoid the changes that will happen to their bodies, and in some instances, the way they think and behave.

Food additives can contribute to a very difficult journey for some young people. I have previously mentioned the teenager in the United Kingdom who is now legally blind and deaf through having a diet of 'junk food' please see page 30: The devils gather. Food additives and junk food can make people sick or very sick. They can also add stress to the mind, brain and body. It's now time to bring the true picture of additives into the public arena.

Food additives and their classification is a minefield to navigate. With the help of some reliable research maybe some light will shine on this subject.

**Types of food additives**

Different types of food additives and their uses:

- **Anti-caking agents** – stop ingredients from becoming lumpy and sticking together.
- **Antioxidants** – prevent foods from oxidising or going rancid.

- **Artificial sweeteners** – increase the sweetness.
- **Emulsifiers** – stop fats from clotting together which allows baking to have an even distribution of ingredients.
- **Food acids** – maintain the right acid level.
- **Colours**- enhance or add colour, from brilliant pink to purple and iridescent greens and garish yellows.
- **Humectants** – keep food moist and allows for a longer shelf life in cakes, bread, rolls and other baked foods bought at the bakery, supermarket and other food outlets.
- **Flavours** – add and enhance flavour.
- **Flavour enhancers** – increase the power and intensity of the flavour.
- **Foaming agents** – maintain uniform and aeration of gases in food and drink. Often seen in cocktails, party cake decoration and other products.
- **Mineral salts** – enhances texture and flavour, can add the 'bite' to some dishes.
- **Preservative** – stops microbes from multiplying and spoiling food.
- **Thickeners and vegetable gum**- enhances texture, consistency and appearance of food.
- **Stabilisers and firming agents** – maintains even ingredient spreading.
- **Flour treatment** – improves baking quality, appearance which increases saleability.

- **Glazing agents** – improves appearance on many foods including chocolates, sweets, confectionary and desserts.
- **Gelling agents** – alter the texture of foods through gel formation and appearance.
- **Propellants** – a gas filled container that helps to propel food from the container.
- **Raising agents or leavening agent** – increases the volume of food through the use of gases, often used in dough products.
- **Bulking agents** – increases the volume of food without major changes to its available energy. These are non-nutritive substances commonly non-starch polysaccharides.
  Topics abstracted and added to: Betterhealth.[61]

## Names to become familiar with

- **Carrier** – a substance used to dissolve, dilute or disperse a food additive or nutrient without altering its function – to improve handling and application.
- **Emulsifier** – an agent that forms or preserves a mixture of substances normally incapable of being mixed, for example: oil and water.
- **Bulking agent** – a filler substance that increases food bulk without increasing available energy.
- **Foaming agent** – facilitates the formation of foam in a liquid or solid food.
- **Glazing agent** – a substance that gives food a shiny appearance or provides a protective coating.

---

[61] https://www.betterhealth.vic.gov.au

- **Gelling agent**- allows the formation of a gel to change food texture.
- **Humectant** – a substance that helps to prevent food from drying out.
- **Sequestrant** – a substance which controls the availability of a cation.[62]
- **Stabiliser** – a substance that maintains a standardized spreading of food, and
- **Thickener** – a substance that increases the viscosity of food.

For more informed information, please go to: https://noshly.com

## Controversial additives

Most of the additives in question are from the following key categories:

- Colours (100 range)
- Preservatives (200 range)
- Antioxidants (300 range)
- Food acids (300 range)
- Mineral salts (300 range)
- Vegetable gums and thickeners (400 range)
- Humectants and artificial sweeteners (400 range)
- Emulsifiers (400 range)
- More mineral salts (400 range)
- Thickeners (400 range)
- More emulsifiers (400 range)
- More mineral salts (500 range)
- Flavour enhancers (600 range)
- Propellants (900 range)
- Artificial sweeteners (900 range)

---

[62] Is a positive charged ion.

- Foaming agents (900 range)
- Additional chemicals and starches (1001 - 1522 range)

**Colours** (code numbers in the 100 range add or restore colour to foods).

Look for the following colour **devils** next time you go to the supermarket to buy your shopping.

**Check:**

- Cakes with coloured icing or toppings
- Drinks with colour
- Biscuits, cakes, and baked bakery goods that have added colour
- Flavoured desserts (milk or otherwise)
- Doughnuts and dough products
- Jellies
- Lollies or sweets (confectionery)
- Ice cream
- Yogurt and
- Jam tarts or jam filled cakes.

And any other food you feel is suspicious.

**Please note:** The symbols used in the following lists may contain: A or α = alpha; β = beta; δ = delta; γ = gamma. Greek letters are commonly used for names of immune-related chemicals.

## Collecting research

While writing this book, my husband and I now walk around the supermarket with added interest. We look closely at the food we buy; I often see him reading labels, something he never did. Some manufacturers are conscious of their brand and want to develop wholesome food. However, there are still those that persist in putting all manner of additives into the product and hope we, the consumer, don't spot the packaging information. Some manufacturers insist on listing their product ingredients in white writing on a light grey background. Or they write the required information so small a telescope is needed to understand what is being said. This is unacceptable and needs to end. We need clear information, in a legible font, preferably with white writing on a royal or dark-blue background. This colour combination is recommended by the Royal Society for the Blind or (RNIB) and is a proven method which allows legibility.

## Additives

Following are over 300 additives. Some of the information may make you angry and upset because the additives used should not be added to any food source in the first place. Some of the information may contribute to your knowledge of a person, who is sick, has been sick and there has been little to no medical information of how and why this person has suffered the way they have of did? You may also answer some of your own questions. It's only by the consumer asking questions will we have the changes needed to make our food safe to eat.

# Becoming aware of the devils

| Safe | Caution | Avoid |
|------|---------|-------|
| 🟢 | 🟠 | 🔴 |

## Devils: Colours (100 range)

| Devil Number | Additive |
|--------------|----------|
| **100**<br>Safe or Caution<br>🟢 🟠 | **Curcumin or turmeric**<br>**(i) (ii)** |

**Colour: Bright yellow – Curcumin or turmeric**

Originally a member of the ginger family. Can be artificially and synthetically produced. Very high doses of synthetic curcumin or turmeric can cause nausea and migraines. Can be high in salicylates,[63] amines[64] or glutamates. In the food industry, maybe made with emulsifiers such as polysorbate 80[65]. Also see 433. Used in ice cream, popcorn, yogurt, cakes, biscuits, gelatine, sauces. There may be intolerance to this product. Check for approval 100, 100(i). Also check if you are buying synthetic or pure Curcumin (turmeric). Medical research and trials seen on the BBC program 'Trust Me I'm A Doctor' show outstanding benefits of pure curcumin. Further research carried out by Dr Sharon McKenna of the Cork Cancer Centre said, *'Scientists have known for a long time that natural compounds have potential to treat faulty cells that have become cancerous and we suspect that curcumin might have therapeutic value.'* She further explained: '*...the team found that curcumin started to kill cancer cells within 24 hours. The*

---

[63] Found in some plants including white willow bark and winter green leaves.

[64] Synthetic: a compound derived from ammonia.

[65] Used as an emulsifier in chocolates and salad dressings.

*cells also began to digest themselves after the curcumin triggered lethal cell death signals.*[66] Approved in the United States, the European Union, New Zealand and Australia. Safe or Caution

| 101 Safe or Caution | Riboflavin(i) (ii) (iii) |
|---|---|

**Colour: Yellow to orange**
Riboflavin (i) is a synthetic. May need further investigation to check source. Naturally found in eggs, cheese, leafy vegetables, liver, kidneys, lean meat, legumes, mushrooms and almonds. Can be genetically modified. Check country approval of (i) (ii) (iii). 101, Approved in the United States, European Union, New Zealand and Australia. Safe or Caution

| 102 Avoid | Tartrazine |
|---|---|

**Colour: Light orange powder or granules**
Is a food colour derived from coal tar.[67] Banned in Norway and Austria. Is used in alcoholic mixtures, beer, breakfast cereals, butter, margarine, chicken broth, chicken cubes, cheeses, sweets, confectionary, crackers, crisps, fizzy drinks, ice cream, frosting, iced lollies, macaroni cheese, flavoured milk, pancake mix, pasta, ready meals with cheese flavouring, yogurt, chewable vitamins. Can cause asthma, hyperactivity in children, depression, anger, behavioural problems, confusion; difficulty in sleeping,

---

[66] http://news.bbc.co.uk
[67] A by-product of coal, coke and coal gas.

concentration problems, learning difficulties, dermatitis and migraine. Severe allergic reactions, including blurred vision. Chronic urticaria, itching and stings to the skin. Can cause Pupura[68] – a disease that causes purple or brownish spots on the skin. Approved in the United States, European Union, New Zealand and Australia. **Avoid**

| 103<br>**Caution** or **Avoid** | **Alkanet** or **Alkannin** |
|---|---|
| **Colour: Yellow to orange**<br>Not allowed in some parts of the Western world. In sensitive asthmatics it may increase a reaction and increase hyperactivity in some children. It may be in the ingredients of medication such as aspirin. On alert in the United States and the European Union. Approval in New Zealand and Australia. **Caution** or **Avoid** ||

| 104<br>**Avoid** | **Quinoline yellow** |
|---|---|
| **Colour: Dull yellow to greenish yellow**<br>Is an artificial coal tar dye used in the production of some food. Found in ices and ice cream, scotch eggs and smoked haddock. May cause dermatitis if used in lipstick manufacture. Also used in hair products and colognes. Commonly used in the United Kingdom. Banned in Germany, Norway, Australia and United States. **Avoid** ||

---

[68] Spots caused by bleeding under the skin – mainly seen in children – seek medical advice.

| 110<br>Caution or Avoid | Sunset yellow FCF |
|---|---|

**Colour: Yellow to orange**
Is a synthetic colour used in cereals, drinks, sweets and confectionary, commercially baked bakery products, snack foods, ice creams and many medications. May have many side effects including: urticaria, (hives), rhinitis (runny nose), hyperactivity, kidney tumours, abdominal pain, nausea, vomiting and indigestion. Banned in Norway. On alert in the United States. Approved in the European Union, New Zealand and Australia. **Caution** or **Avoid**

| 120<br>Caution or Avoid | Cochineal or carmines or carmic acid |
|---|---|

**Colour: Deep red**
Extracted from the crushed carcasses of the female Dactylopius coccus scale insect. Used in alcoholic drinks with calcium carmine in insoluble form. Is used in a number of products including: commercially baked breads and bakery products, toppings, biscuits, desserts, drinks, icings, pie fillings, some varieties of cheddar cheese and sauces, sweets and confectionary. Can cause allergies, hyper-sensitive reactions, asthma, gastrointestinal disorders, skin ailments, eczema, dermatitis, itching and hives. On alert in the United States. Approved in the European Union, New Zealand and Australia. **Caution** or **Avoid**

| 122 Avoid | Azorubine or carmoisine C114720 |
|---|---|

**Colour: red to maroon**

Azorubine (Carmoisine). Synthetic food dye of the azo[69] food group and derivative of coal tar. Can produce severe reactions in asthmatics. Is used in confectionary, jelly crystals and marzipan. Suspected carcinogen, mutagen, skin rashes, oedema, hyperactivity in some people. United Kingdom is evaluating health risks. Banned in Canada, Japan, Sweden, Austria and Norway. On alert in the United States. Approved in the European Union, New Zealand and Australia. **Avoid**

| 123 Avoid | Amaranth |
|---|---|

**Colour: Purple to red (blackcurrant)**

Is a synthetic azo dye derived from coal tar. Found in ice cream, jams, jelly, tinned fruit, pie fillings, trifles, prawns and in gravy granules. May cause skin rash and skin disorders. Intolerance to asthmatics and can provoke eczema and hyperactivity in some children. It may cause birth defects and has caused foetal defects in some animal testing. Possibility of a link to cancer. Not recommended for children. Banned in Russia, Austria, Norway and restricted to caviar in France and Italy. On alert in the United States. Approved in the European Union, New Zealand and Australia. **Avoid**

---

[69] Azo compounds have vivid colours, especially reds, oranges, and yellows.

| 124<br>**Avoid** | Ponceau 4R |
|---|---|

**Colour: Brilliant red**
Is an artificial, synthetic food colour used to add a tint of red to strawberry juice, colour dessert toppings, colour salami, fruit pie fillings, cake mixes, truffles, soups and added to sweets and confectionary. Will cause allergies, hyper-sensitive reactions, asthma, behavioural problems, hyperactivity and learning difficulties. Also *'linked to atrophy of the adrenaline glands, bladder polyps, cancer and urticaria.'[70]* Banned in Canada, Norway, restricted in Sweden. On alert in the United States. Approved in New Zealand and Australia. **Avoid**

| 127<br>**Avoid** | Erythrosine |
|---|---|

**Colour: Cherry-pink/red**
A synthetic coal tar dye found in cocktail glacé and tinned cherries, canned fruit, custard mix, sweets, bakery, snack foods, biscuits, chocolate, dressed crab, garlic sausage, luncheon meat, salmon spread, pâté, scotch eggs, stuffed olives and packet trifle mix. Could affect thyroid activity, can increase hormone levels and lead to hyperthyroidism. Implicated in phototoxicity (sensitivity to light). May produce hyperactivity in children. Not recommended for children. May be linked to brain dysfunction, thyroid abnormality and cancer. Banned in Norway. On alert in the United States. Approved in the European Union, New Zealand and Australia. **Avoid**

---

[70] http://thearticlebay.com

| 129 **Avoid** | Allura red AC |
|---|---|

**Colour: Orange to red**
Used in many sweets, confectionery, drinks, condiments, medications. Also used in biscuits, dairy products, fruit flavoured fillings, gelatine, cake mixes and puddings, Not recommended for child consumption. Severe reaction by asthmatics and people intolerant to aspirin. Linked to cancer in laboratory animals. Banned in Denmark, Belgium, France, Germany, Switzerland, Sweden, Austria and Norway. On alert in the United States. Approved in the European Union, New Zealand and Australia. **Avoid**

| 132 **Avoid** | Indigotine |
|---|---|

**Colour: Blue**
Blue synthetic coal tar dye, normally produced by synthesis of indoxyl in which a molecule is bound to another functional group by fusion of sodium phenylglycinate in a mixture of caustic soda and sodamide.[71] Added to tablets and capsules and used in ice cream, sweets, confectionary, baked foods, biscuits. Allergy sufferers should avoid this product. So too, should people with skin conditions, blood pressure or breathing problems. Not recommended for consumption by children. Banned in Norway. On alert in the United States. Approved the European Union, New Zealand and Australia. **Avoid**

---

[71] White compound, crystalline dehydrating agent.

| 133 | Brilliant blue FCF |
|---|---|
| **Avoid** | |

**Colour: Blue powder or granules**

Aluminium solution or ammonium salts. Is an artificial food colouring used to make candy floss, (cotton candy), ice cream, canned and processed peas, blueberry flavoured products, dairy products, sweets, icings for cakes, children's ice blocks, drinks, confectionary and mouthwash. Asthmatics avoid. Suspected of being a carcinogen. Linked to hyperactivity. On alert in the United States. Approved in the European Union, New Zealand and Australia. **Avoid**

| 140 | Chlorophyll |
|---|---|
| **Safe** or **Caution** | |

**Colour: Green**

A natural colour within all plants and algae. May be extracted by the use of dangerous solvents (check extraction method). Safe chlorophyll is extracted as a food additive from grasses, nettles and alfalfa. **Safe** or **Caution**

| 141 Caution | Chlorophyll-copper complex Chlorophyll copper complexes 141(i) Chlorophyll copper complexes potassium and sodium 141(ii) |
|---|---|

**Colour: Natural olive green**

Contains sodium and potassium salts (concentrated natural colours can be high in salicylates,[72] amines or glutamates.'[73] May be extracted with dangerous solvents. Dangerous to people who are sensitive to copper. Approved in the United States, European Union, New Zealand and Australia. **Caution**

| 142 Avoid | Green S |
|---|---|

**Colour: Green**

A green synthetic coal tar dye found in gravy and gravy granules, desserts, ice cream, mint sauce, packet breadcrumbs, tinned peas and cake mixes. Will cause hyperactivity in children and adults. Causes asthma, urticaria (inflamed reddened patches on the skin), depression, anger, difficulty in sleeping, difficulty in concentrating, especially in children. Banned in Canada, Finland, Japan, Norway and Sweden. On alert in the United States. Approved in the European Union, New Zealand and Australia. **Avoid**

---

[72] In severe cases, a salicylate allergy can lead to anaphylaxis. https://www.webmd.com

[73] https://www.fedup.com.au

| 143 Avoid | Fast green FCF |
|---|---|

**Colour: Red to violet powder or crystals**

Is an organic salt which is poorly absorbed by the intestines. Used in tinned green peas and other vegetables, jellies, sauces, fish, desserts and dry bakery products. Has proven to promote tumours and mutations in animal experiments. Concentrated levels will cause eye irritation and possible digestive respiratory tract irritation, asthma and allergic reactions. The use of this food dye is prohibited in some countries. On alert in the United States and the European Union. Approved in New Zealand and Australia. Avoid

| 150a Avoid | Caramel I |
|---|---|

**Colour: Red to yellow**

Produced from sugar and glucose. May be made from genetically modified starches. Is plain caramel, caustic with a dark-brown odourless liquid. Has a strong aftertaste, is stable in alcohol, tannin and salt enriched environments. Used in soy, fruit and canned sauces, beer, whiskey, cola, biscuits and pickles. May cause gastrointestinal and liver problems. Linked to: '*birth defects, neurological disorders, negative effects on the immune system, decrease in white blood cells and convulsions.*'[74] Approved in the United States, European Union, New Zealand and Australia. Avoid

---

[74] http://thearticlebay.com

| 150b **Avoid** | Caramel II **Sulfite caramel** |
|---|---|

**Colour: Red tones**
Caustic sulphite caramel is made from sucrose in the presence of ammonia, ammonium sulphate, sulphur dioxide or sodium hydroxide. Mild flavour and aroma, stabile in alcohol. Used in tea, wine, rum, whiskey, brandy, cognac, sherry, some vinegar, light cake mixes and other snack foods. Will cause asthma in some people. Causes hyperactivity, gastrointestinal conditions, liver problems and linked to: *'birth defects, neurological disorders, negative effects on the immune system, decrease in white blood cells, convulsions.'*[75] Approved in the United States, European Union, New Zealand, Australia. **Avoid**

| 150c **Avoid** | Caramel III **Ammonia process** |
|---|---|

**Colour: Red-brown to black**
Can be made from genetically modified crops. Ammonia caramel, baker's caramel, confectioner's caramel, beer caramel. Stable in alcohol and salt-rich environments. Used in beer, cereals, pet food, liquorice, confectionery, gravy, soy and BBQ sauce. Will cause hyperactivity, gastrointestinal conditions, liver problems, reproductive problems. Is linked to: *'birth defects, neurological disorders, negative effects on the immune system, decrease in white blood cells, convulsions.'* See 150b above. Also linked to attention deficit hyperactivity disorder (ADHD). Approved in the United States, European Union, New Zealand and Australia. **Avoid**

---

[75] http://thearticlebay.com

| 150d **Avoid** | Caramel IV Ammonia sulphite process |
|---|---|

**Colour: Rich dark brown**

Known as 4-Mel is a sulfite ammonia. Acid-proof caramel used in many drink and food products. Stable in alcohol, tannin and acid-rich environments. Used in soft and fizzy drinks and other carbonated beverages, balsamic vinegar, coffee, chocolate syrups, baked goods, cocoa extenders, pet food, sauces, soy sauce, soups, meat rubs, seasoning blends, beer, biscuits, cakes, chocolate, confectionary, sweets and lollies, crisps, doughnuts, flour products, fruit sauces, ice cream, pickles, oyster sauce, pâté, preserves, soy sauce, whiskey, wine, meat and vegetable substitutes. Is known to cause asthma, hyperactivity, hypersensitivity, gastrointestinal disorder and liver problems. Carbohydrates and ammonia are used to produce caramel.

The Centre for Science in the Public Interest (CSPI). '... *the FDA immediately should change the name 'caramel colouring' to 'chemically modified caramel colouring' or 'ammonia-sulfite process caramel colouring' and should not allow products to be labelled 'natural' if they contain any type of caramel colouring.'*[76] Is linked to asthma, hyperactivity, hypersensitivity, gastrointestinal conditions, liver problems. Also linked to: *'birth defects, neurological disorders, negative effects on the immune system, decrease in white blood cells, convulsions.'*[77] See 150b. Also causes vitamin B deficiency. Approved in the United States, European Union, New Zealand and Australia. **Avoid**

---

[76] http://www.befoodsmart.com Source: Centre for Science in the Public Interest.

[77] http://thearticlebay.com

| 151 **Avoid** | Brilliant black BN or Brilliant black PN |
|---|---|

**Colour: Black powder or granules**
Is a synthetic, black tar derivative used in brown sauces, black current cake mixes, food decorations and coatings, sweets, some confectionery, jams, fish paste and soft drinks. Is linked to asthma, gastrointestinal conditions, hyperactivity, skin conditions: eczema, linked dermatitis, hives and linked to cancer. Is on alert in the United States, Belgium, Germany, Switzerland, Japan, Finland and Sweden. Approved in the European Union, New Zealand and Australia. **Avoid**

| 153 **Avoid** | Carbons black or Vegetable carbon |
|---|---|

**Colour: Black odourless powder**
Is black in colour derived from vegetable carbon. Used in many liquorice products, sweets, confectionary, jams and some health foods. May increase hyperactivity in children. Can contribute to allergies. May contribute to skin ailments including eczema, dermatitis and hives. Is linked to cancer. Is also described as natural colour. If not derived from vegetable products may also be derived from animal parts. On alert in the United States. Approved in the European Union, New Zealand and Australia. **Avoid**

| 155 Avoid | Brown HT also called chocolate brown HT C1 52028 |
|---|---|

**Colour: Brown**

Is a brown synthetic coal tar diazo dye.[78] Used to substitute cocoa or caramel as a colorant. Used in chocolate cakes, milk, cheeses, jams, yogurts, ice cream, fruit products, fish and other products. Can cause allergic reactions and induce skin sensitivity. May cause asthma, gastrointestinal problems, dermatitis and hives. The Hyperactive Children's Support Group recommends eliminating it from the diet of children. Banned in Austria, Belgium, Denmark, France, Germany Norway and Sweden. On alert in the United States. Approved in the European Union, New Zealand and Australia. **Avoid**

| 160a Caution or Avoid | Carotene |
|---|---|

**Colour: yellow to orange**

Carotene is either natural or synthetic. In natural food colour is isolated from several plants. The body converts natural carotene to vitamin A in the liver. Synthetic carotene is extracted by the dangerous solvent hexane[79] and has been proven to cause birth defects and to increase the risk of cancer and death rates among smokers.

---

[78] Diazo dyes contain chemical groups that bind metal ions together, chromium and copper being the most popular. Used widely in cotton and silk dying.

[79] Hexane is an organic compound made of carbon and hydrogen commonly isolated as a by-product of petroleum and crude oil refinement. Is used in as a chemical extractor in the food industry.

Approved in the United States, European Union, New Zealand and Australia. **Caution** or **Avoid**

| 160c **Caution** or **Avoid** | Paprica |
|---|---|

**Colour: Red to orange**
Also known as capsanthian or capsorubin. Is a natural food extract that can be extracted through dangerous solvents. May be linked to cancer. Is banned in many countries. Approved in the United States, European Union, New Zealand and Australia. **Caution** or **Avoid**

| 160d **Caution** | Lycopene |
|---|---|

**Colour: Bright red**
Can be extracted using dangerous solvents. Found in tomatoes and other red fruits and vegetables including carrots, watermelons and papayas. Natural Lycopene has been proven to be a powerful anti-cancer agent. If possible, check for extraction methods. Approved in the United States, European Union and New Zealand. Check for approval in Australia. **Caution**

| 160e **Caution** or **Avoid** | Betta-apo-8'-Carotenal (30) |
|---|---|

**Colour: Orange-red to yellow**
Could be synthetic derived from beta-carotene through the use of dangerous solvents. If extracted with hexane, it may

cause severe sickness including hexane poisoning. Is used as a food colour in some cheeses, including sliced cheeses. Also used in fat-based commercial products, salad dressings, margarine, sauces, dairy products, beverages, sweets, lollies or confectionary. May cause endocrine disturbance. On alert in the United States. Approved in the European Union. Approved in New Zealand and Australia. **Caution** or **Avoid**

| 160f **Caution** or **Avoid** | Betta-apo-8' Carotenoic acid, methyl or ethyl ester (30) |
|---|---|

**Colour: Orange-red to yellow**
May be a synthetic colour extracted from beta-carotene with dangerous solvents, including hexane. Has caused endocrine disturbance. On alert in the United States. Approved in the European Union, New Zealand and Australia. **Caution** or **Avoid**

| 161a **Caution** or **Avoid** | Flavoxanthin |
|---|---|

**Colour: Golden yellow**
May contain salicylates,[80] amines[81] or glutamates. Are found in small quantities in a variety of plants. May cause headaches. On alert in the United States and the European Union. Approved in New Zealand and Australia. **Caution** or **Avoid**

---

[80] Salicylates occur naturally in plants.
[81] An organic compound derived from ammonia.

177

| 161b<br>**Caution** or **Avoid** | Lutein |
|---|---|

**Colour: Orange-red to yellow**
Naturally found in green leaves, marigolds, egg yolks, kale and spinach. May be extracted through the use of dangerous chemicals. May cause brain damage and damage to the kidneys, reproductive organs and nervous system. On
alert in the United States. Approved in the European Union, New Zealand and Australia. **Caution** or **Avoid**

| 161c<br>**Caution** | Kryptoxanthin or Cryptoxanthin |
|---|---|

**Colour: Dark-reddish brown**
Is extracted from plants, the petals of flowers, orange rind, papaya, egg yolk, butter, apples and bovine blood serum. Can be used in sweets and confectionary. On alert in the United States and in the European Union. Approved in New Zealand and Australia. **Caution**

| 161d<br>**Caution** | Rubixanthin |
|---|---|

**Colour: Yellow**
Usually extracted from rose hips. Can be extracted with hexane, a dangerous food extractor. On alert in the United States and in the European Union. Approved in New Zealand and Australia. **Caution**

| 161e<br>**Caution** or **Avoid** | Violoxanthin |
|---|---|

**Colour: Orange**
A food additive and colouring derived from a number of different plants, including pansies. Check for method of extraction. May contain salicylates,[82] amines and glutamates. On alert in the United States and the European Union. Approved in New Zealand and Australia. **Caution** or **Avoid**

| 161f<br>**Caution** or **Avoid** | Rhodoxanthin |
|---|---|

**Colour: Purple**
Is found in small quantities in a variety of plants and some bird feathers. Can be high in salicylates, amines and glutamates. On alert in the United States and the European Union. Approved in New Zealand and Australia. **Caution** or **Avoid**

| 162<br>**Avoid** | Beet red |
|---|---|

**Colour: Deep-red purple**
A natural extract from beetroot. Can be used in burgers, ice cream, jellies, desserts, liquorice, oxtail soup, sauces, sweets and confectionary. Not suitable for infants and small children. May be linked to 'birth defects, poisoning,

---

[82] A salt or ester of salicylic acid.

*genetic damage, methemoglobinemia, (blood disorder), sudden death, tumours, cancer, severe allergic reaction.'*[83] Also see Potassium 249. On alert in the United States. Approved in the European Union, New Zealand and Australia. **Avoid**

| 163<br>**Safe** or **Caution** | Anthocyanins<br>or<br>Grape skin or<br>blackcurrent extract<br>(iv) (v) |
|---|---|

**Colour: Deep-purple, red or green**
Derived from plants and flowers. Used as colouring in dairy products, soups, glacé cherries, sweets, lollies and confectionary. Also used in pickles, soft drinks, ice cream, black cherry yogurt, tomato and vegetable soups. Safe if extracted without the use of hexane. On alert in the Unites States. 163 (iv) and 163 (v). On alert in the European Union, New Zealand and Australia. **Safe** or **Caution**

| 164<br>**Caution** or **Avoid** | Saffron or Crocetin or<br>crocin, also known as<br>gardenia yellow |
|---|---|

**Colour: Red to orange**
May be mixed with synthetic or artificial colour. Can cause allergies and have a hypersensitive reaction with some people. Approved in the United States. On alert in the European union. Approved in New Zealand and Australia. **Caution** or **Avoid**

---

[83] http://thearticlebay.com

| 170 Caution or Avoid | Calcium carbonate also calcium carbonate (i) and (ii) |
|---|---|

**Colour: White mineral salt**
Used as white in colouring. Used in toothpaste, white paint and cleaning powders. May contain high levels of lead. Used in tinned vegetables and fruit. Also used in commercial production to make bread, cakes and flour products, including wines. High doses may contribute to mineral imbalances in the human body. Can also contribute to confused behaviour, haemorrhoids, kidney stones, abdominal pain, constipation, anal bleeding and fissures. Approved in the United States, European Union, New Zealand and Australia. **Caution** or **Avoid**

| 171 Avoid | Titanium dioxide |
|---|---|

**Colour: White**
Used in vitamin supplements, sauces, cheeses, cakes and biscuits. Also used in confectionary and in pure white icing. Not environmentally friendly as it may pollute waterways. Recent animal studies have shown that high concentrations have caused respiratory tract and lung cancer in rats. Is used in toothpaste and for food whitening. Is linked to *'cell death, blocking of cell communication, negative effects on the immune system, mutations, cancer, heart problems, severe allergic reactions.'*[84] Approved in the United States, European Union, New Zealand and Australia. **Avoid**

---

[84] http://thearticlebay.com

| 172<br>Caution or Avoid | Iron oxid<br>also iron oxide<br>(i) (ii) (iii) |
|---|---|

**Colour: Red, black and yellow mineral colours**
Used to colour capsules and health food vitamins also used in herbal supplements. Used to colour sausage skins in the production of sausages. Can be found in cake and dessert mixes, tinned fish, including salmon and shrimp paste. Also used in meat paste. Is also used in some manufactured soup products. Does not chemically degrade in the human body. Leads to possible kidney damage, is suspect as a neurotoxin. Has lead to blindness in dog studies. Approved in the United States, European Union, New Zealand and Australia. Caution or Avoid

| 173<br>Avoid | Aluminium |
|---|---|

**Colour: silver grey**
There is no dietary requirement within the human body for this additive. Is used in sugar-coated and flour confectionary decorations and in the presentation of dragées (small bite-sized confectionary with a hard, external shell). May be used in other foods and drinks. Is linked to premature senility, Parkinson's and Alzheimer's disease, osteoporosis, some kidney disease; toxicity of the nervous system, cardiovascular system, the reproductive and respiratory systems. Banned in some countries. On alert in the United States. Approved in the European Union, New Zealand and Australia. Avoid

| 174 **Avoid** | Silver |
|---|---|

**Colour: Silver**

Is used as a colouring agent in food and drink products. Is used as a decoration on sugar-coated and flour products. Also used for cake and chocolate decorations and in the presentation of dragées (small bite-sized confectionary with a hard, external shell). May change skin colour to a bluish-green colour. Linked to kidney damage and disease, lung damage, gastrointestinal irritation and some poisoning. Banned in some countries. Approved in the United States,
European Union. Check for approval in New Zealand. Was banned in Australia prior to 1999. Now approved in Australia. **Avoid**

| 175 **Avoid** | Gold |
|---|---|

**Colour: Gold**

Gold has no dietary requirements within the human body. Is used for cake and chocolate decorations and in the presentation of dragées (small bite-sized confectionary with a hard, external shell). Is used as a colouring in cake decoration. Is linked to: '*blood production in bone marrow, cancer, severe allergic reactions and accumulates in the kidneys.*'[85] Banned in some countries. On alert in the United States. Approved in the European Union, New Zealand and Australia. **Avoid**

---

[85] http://thearticlebay.com

| 180 **Avoid** | Lithol rupine BK |
|---|---|

**Colour: Red to brown**
Is an azo dye[86] used in cotton and silk dying. Is a dangerous food colour and additive derived from coal tar and petroleum. Used in cheese rind. May cause severe allergic reactions in asthmatics and hyperactivity in children. Is banned in some countries. On alert in the United States. Approved in the European Union. On alert in New Zealand and Australia. **Avoid**

| 181 **Caution** or **Avoid** | Tannic acid Tannins |
|---|---|

**Colour: Yellowish white to light brown**
Can be either natural or synthetic. May be prepared from acorns, nut galls, twigs and bark of oak trees. Is naturally in many caffeine drinks including tea and coffee. Large doses are associated with gastric irritation and liver damage. Approved in the United States. On alert in the European Union. Approved in New Zealand and Australia. **Caution** or **Avoid**

Please see Chapter Three, page 139 – synthetic caffeine.

It's not until we've eaten something that has had a reaction on our bodily system or witnessed seeing our loved one's in pain or seen the reaction of children to different foods that we start to question the ingredients

---

[86] Any of a large class of synthetic dyes whose molecules contain two adjacent nitrogen atoms between carbon atoms.

of the food, drink or confectionary we or they have consumed.

It's through watching and experiencing, not only the children in the classroom but with my own family that I really began to question the validity of the food stuff I was buying. Having carried out this research it is now opening my eyes to '**the not so good**' products on the supermarket shelves. Having said that, there are some very good products to buy but the bad products need to be eliminated so the temptation to buy products with glitzy marketing and packaging are removed. As we get older, when walking around the supermarket, we sometimes reminisce about childhood favourite foods and then we buy! The product in question may be full of undesirable ingredients but the pressure to buy because of our memories and emotions can become difficult to resist. As you will see, there are many preservatives in everyday, favourite foods.

## My story of 252 potassium nitrate and 319 tert-Butylhydroquinone (TBHQ)

Hindsight is a great educator. It was one of those autumn days and when living in Berkshire, United Kingdom, I had arranged to meet some friends at Reading, Railway Station; we were going into London to meet another friend and then go on to see a live, daytime show in the West End. As we were planning our return trip back to Australia, I thought it would be a brilliant day's outing. These rare opportunities would not come about so frequently once the 'big move' was made.

Having travelled into London by train, we met our friend at a Chinese restaurant in the heart of London and not far from the theatre. We had an OK meal; I must admit I didn't feel very well after eating the food. We then went to the theatre to enjoy the show, which was amazing. On the train and on the journey back to Reading, I felt not so good, however, my friends had bought fast take away meals at Paddington Station and sat on the train eating, chatting and enjoying their 'junk food'.

I arrived home late that night. I started to feel a bit better the following day. On day two I remember getting up from the chair and suddenly my head would spin this would result in feeling sick and then the dizziness would start. I would need to sit down and take a breath, collect my thoughts while I restabilised how I felt and then try to get up again. Eventually, if I kept my head straight and didn't move my body too fast, I could get the jobs done I needed to do and would feel OK as long as I didn't move my head quickly or too sharply.

The episodes of vertigo and the feeling of sickness would last up to ten or fifteen minutes. Eventually, the vertigo passed but then the ringing in the ears started. Yes, it was Tinnitus and I have been living with this condition for the last nine or so years.

I'm near the completion of the book and have researched a great deal on food additives and have been shocked by my findings.

Starting out and at the beginning of the writing for this book, it was not my goal to research the topic of Tinnitus and I cannot correlate vertigo, tinnitus and the food additives 252, potassium nitrate and 319 tert-Butylhydroquinone (TBHQ) together. But I did not have any form of dizziness, sickness before the Asian meal in London.

As my research goes on and now with the discovery that 252, potassium nitrate does contribute to vertigo and 319 (TBHQ) contributes to the long-term condition of Tinnitus, there are questions, I need to ask and as a consumer, I need to have answers.

**How much of the above additives are needed in a single meal to make a person sick?**

**Your Notes**

..............................................................................

..............................................................................

..............................................................................

..............................................................................

..............................................................................

..............................................................................

..............................................................................

..............................................................................

..............................................................................

..............................................................................

..............................................................................

..............................................................................

..............................................................................

..............................................................................

..............................................................................

..............................................................................

..............................................................................

..............................................................................

# Devils: Preservatives (200 range)

| Devil Numbers | Additive |
|:---:|:---:|
| **200**<br>Avoid | **Sorbic acid** |

**Colour: Free flowing colourless needles of powder**
In smaller quantities occurs in fruit. Synthetic produced by additive industry and used in sweet wine making, processed and non-processed cheese, cider, dessert sauces, soft drinks, sweets or lollies and confectionary, yogurt, soup concentrates, candied peel, fermented dairy products, fruit salads, lemonade and ades, pizza, rye bread, cakes and bakery products, lemon juice, shellfish and medicines. If sensitive, can cause skin irritation, asthmatics should avoid. Is linked to hyperactivity and behavioural problems. Can cause skin conditions: eczema, dermatitis, itching and hives. Is linked to cancer and liver damage. Approved for use in the United States, European Union, New Zealand and Australia. **Avoid**

| | |
|:---:|:---:|
| **201**<br>Avoid | **Sodium sorbate** |

**Colour: White salt of sorbic acid**
A commercially produced, synthetic food preservative used in: dried apricots, candied peel, cheese, cider, fermented milks, pie fillings and toppings, fruit salads, gelatine capsules, frozen pizzas, margarine, processed cheese, cheese spreads and cheese slices, soft drinks, soup concentrates, yogurts and sweets. Is also used in sauces, cheesecake mixes, pickled cucumbers, pineapple juice, salad dressings, soya sauce, table olives and preserved prawns. Causes headaches, intestinal damage and upset,

constipation, asthma, liver damage and is linked to (ADHD).[87] Approved in the United States. On alert in the European Union. Approved in New Zealand and Australia. **Avoid**

| 202 **Avoid** | Potassium sorbate |
|---|---|

**Colour: White to yellow crystals or crystalline granules**
A synthetic additive used in pie fillings and toppings, concentrated fruit juices, cheeses, fermented milks, fruit salads, gelatine capsules, jams and preserves, glacé cherries, fruit salads, cheese spreads, cheese slices, seafood dressings, soft drinks, wine, yogurt, pickled cucumbers, margarine and salad dressings. Causes skin irritation, contributes to asthma and hyperactivity, ADHD, diarrhoea, vomiting, stomach or intestinal pain, headaches, liver damage, may create genetic damage. Approved in the United States, European Union, New Zealand and Australia. **Avoid**

| 203 **Avoid** | Calcium sorbate |
|---|---|

**Colour: White crystalline powder**
Is a chemical preservative used in jams, soft drink, meat, cider, concentrated fruit juice, dried apricots, fermented milks, frozen pizzas, fruit salads, margarine, processed and sliced cheeses, salad dressings, table olives, wine, yogurt, glacé cherries, sweets, lollies and confectionary.

---

[87] Attention Deficit Hyperactive Disorder (ADHD).

Contributes to ADHD. Aggravates and contributes to behavioural problems, asthma attacks and allergic reactions. Causes skin irritation, dermatitis, itching and hives. Not recommended for children. Approved in the United States. Now banned in the European Union.[88] Approved in New Zealand and Australia. **Avoid**

| 210 **Avoid** | Benzoic acid |
|---|---|

**Colour: Colourless crystalline solid**
In its natural state is available from berries, fruit and vegetables. Benzoin is a resin exuded from native Asian trees. Used in margarine, cheeses, fruit juice and fruit juice pulp, jam, pickles, salad creams, salad dressing, yogurt, frozen dairy products, soft confectionary and sweets, chewing gum, cordial and fruit drinks, condiments, sugar substitutes, some marinated fish, baked goods, flavouring syrups and some cough medications. Also added to frozen dairy products, relishes, soft sweets and lollies, cordials, and alcohol. Can cause hyperactivity in children. May react with asthmatics and people who suffer from allergies. Can cause headaches, damage to intestinal microbiota and constipation. Is linked to *'birth defects, brain damage, neurological disorders, cell mutations, testicular cancer, asthma, severe allergic reactions, chronic urticaria, dermatitis, delayed growth.'*[89] On alert in the United States. Approved in the European Union. Not approved in New Zealand and Australia. **Avoid**

---

[88] https://www.foodnavigator.com
[89] http://thearticlebay.com

| 211<br>**Avoid** | **Sodium benzoate** |
|---|---|

**Colour: White crystalline powder, flakes or granules**
Is a chemical and synthetic preservative used as an antiseptic to stop food spoilage. Also used to disguise the taste of poor quality, manufactured food products. Helps to protect food against micro-organisms. Can occur naturally in fresh fruit. Used in table olives, syrups, fruit juices, pickles, sauces, jams, carbonated drinks, vinegar, salad dressings, milk, meat products and salads. May cause skin rash, skin issues, asthma attacks and behavioural problems. Also linked to learning difficulties, ADHD and hyperactivity. Has been related to cancer. Also linked to: *'birth defects, neurological disorders, cell mutations, testicular cancer and Parkinson's disease.'*[90] Not recommended for children. Approved for use in the United States, European Union, New Zealand and Australia. **Avoid**

| 212<br>**Avoid** | **Potassium benzoate** |
|---|---|

**Colour: White crystalline powder**
Is a synthetic preservative. Inhibits bacteria and mould in manufactured food and beverage products. Used in margarine, pickled cucumbers, marinated table olives, barbeque sauce, cheesecake mixes, prawns, maple syrup, salad dressings, soy sauce, milk and some milk products, relishes, condiments, soft drinks, baked goods, confectionary, sweets, lollies, minced fruit pies and pineapple juice. Asthmatics should avoid. May produce nettle rash or like rashes, also behavioural problems,

---

[90] http://thearticlebay.com

hyperactivity, depression, difficulty in sleeping for children and adults and hormone imbalance. On alert in the United States. Approved in the European Union, New Zealand and Australia. **Avoid**

| 213<br>Avoid | Calcium benzoate |
|---|---|

**Colour: White crystal powder**
A food additive used in fighting yeast mould and bacteria. Commonly used in fruit juice, soy milk and soy milk drinks, soy sauce, vinegar, bread making and bakery products, also used in cheesecake mix, prawns, pickled cucumbers, relishes and sauces, baked goods, sweets, confectionary, lollies and mouth wash. Also used as a spray fertiliser. Can aggravate allergies, asthmatic conditions, skin ailments, itching, hives and rashes. May have other and more severe reactions. Is linked to: *'…birth defects increased significantly in combination with aspirin, brain damage, neurological disorders, cell mutations, testicular cancer, chronic urticaria, dermatitis and delayed growth.'*[91] Not recommended for consumption by children. On alert in the United States. Approved in the European Union, New Zealand and Australia. **Avoid**

| 216<br>Caution or Avoid | Sodium propyl<br>p-hydroxybenzoate |
|---|---|

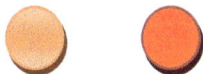

**Colour: White crystalline powder**
Traditionally found in fresh fruit, especially cranberries, mushrooms and some dairy products. Used to protect food from deterioration. In commercial and mass production

---

[91] http://thearticlebay.com

this synthetic powder is used in beer making, fruit sauces, preserves, fruit desserts, fruit cordials and juices. May leave numbness in the mouth; can lead to dermatitis or eczema. May cause problems for asthmatics or people who are sensitive to aspirin. May contribute to skin ailments: itching and soreness, dermatitis, hives and rashes. Not suitable for children or infants. Approved in the United States. On alert in the European Union. Approved in the New Zealand and Australia. Caution or Avoid

| 218 Avoid | Methylparaben or Methyl-p-hydroxybenzoate |
|---|---|

**Colour: White crystalline powder or colourless crystals** Is used as a preservative in baked goods, alcoholic drinks, ice cream, medicines and medications. Often added to milk, including cheese, and meat products. Also added to margarine, pickled cucumbers, some manufactured fruit products, pickles, sauces, soft drinks, table olives, pineapple juice, processed fish and desserts. May contribute to numbing of the mouth or tongue. Children may have difficulty in concentrating after eating products containing this preservative. Difficulty in sleeping, depression, anger, migraine, hormone disruption, eczema, rash, gastrointestinal ailments, asthma, itching and possible skin irritation or reactions. Approved in the United States, European Union, New Zealand and Australia. Avoid

| 220 Avoid | Sulphur dioxide |
|---|---|

**Colour: A strong pungent gas**

A preservative obtained from coal tar. Is produced by the combustion of sulphur and gypsum. In the United States, the use of this product is prohibited on fresh fruit and vegetables. Used in wine making and for preservation of dried prunes, apricots, raisins and dried fruits. Found in beer, juices, cordials, vinegar and prepared potato products. Used as a bleaching agent in flour. Reduces absorption of vitamin B1 and other B vitamins. May cause wheezing in asthmatics, difficulty in breathing if you aren't asthmatic, facial swelling or hive type skin reactions. Is difficult to metabolize for people with impaired kidney function. Is linked to: *'birth defects, genetic damage, nerve damage, behavioural disorders in children, unconsciousness, seizures, swelling in the brain, vomiting, visual disturbance and severe allergic reactions. Approximately 30-40 people die each year in the United States because of 220 – 228.*[92] Not recommended for babies or young children. Approved in the United States, European Union, New Zealand and Australia. **Avoid**

| 221 Avoid | Sodium sulphite, sulfite |
|---|---|

**Colour: White powder with a faint odour of sulphur dioxide**

Is a sulphite decontaminating agent used in fresh orange juice. Sulphites are added to many fruit drinks, sausages, dried fruits, fresh fruits and vegetables, beer, wine, fruit juices, sauces, frozen shellfish, bread, egg yolk products,

---

[92] http://thearticlebay.com

caramel, salads, and other foods. They destroy vitamin B1, B12 and vitamin E. Used to protect food and beverages from microorganisms and oxidation. May cause severe reactions in asthmatics, cause headaches, migraine, intestinal upset, skin disorders and ailments, eczema and dermatitis; creates behavioural problems, can contribute to ADHD, cause gastric irritation and nausea. Approved in the United States, European Union, New Zealand and Australia. **Avoid**

| 222<br>**Avoid** | **Sodium hydrogen bisulphite, (bisulfite)** |
|---|---|

**Colour: Clear to white crystals**
Synthetic preservative used in beer and wine making. Also used as a preservative in preserving cod, sugar, corn syrup, quick frozen potato and quick frozen mashed potato products, milk and milk products, fruit and vegetable juices, fresh fruit and vegetables, puddings, custards, baked goods, bread, soft drinks, sauces, condiments and relish. Destroys vitamin B1 and E. Sometimes used in disinfectants. May cause allergic reaction in asthmatics and allergic reactions and hyper-sensitivity, headaches, migraine, irritating skin conditions including eczema, dermatitis, itching, hives and rashes. Is linked to: '*birth defects, genetic damage, nerve damage, severe breathing difficulties, especially in asthmatics, behavioural disorder, especially in children, unconsciousness, seizures, swelling in the brain, vomiting, visual disturbances, intestinal inflammation, nausea, rash and severe allergic reactions.*'[93] May cause low blood pressure and anaphylactic shock. Not recommended for child consumption. On alert in the United States. Approved in the European Union, New Zealand and Australia. **Avoid**

---

[93] http://thearticlebay.com

196

| 223 Avoid | Sodium metabisulphate |
|-----------|------------------------|

**Colour: White crystals or crystalline powder – has an odour of sulphur dioxide**

Is used as a flour bleaching agent, preservative, disinfectant and antioxidant. Is used in beer and wine making. Also used in sausages, dried raisins, dates, apples, frozen vegetables, vinegar, apple cider vinegar, fruit concentrate juices, concentrated tomato juice, cereal, muesli, cracker biscuits, paste, pulp, puree, canned vegetables and fruits, frozen French fries, fruit syrups, fruit fillings, marmalade, jellies, sugar syrups, pickled condiments, coleslaw, sauerkraut, mustard, relish, ketchup, soy products, (tofu), snack foods, dried spices, herbs, tea, processed potatoes, shell and fish products, fresh grapes, glazed and glace fruits. Not recommended for children. Can cause respiratory reactions in asthmatics. May cause gastric irritation and intestinal discomfort. Contributes to nettle rash, swelling and skin reactions including: eczema, dermatitis, itching, hives and rashes. Can cause behavioural problems; contribute to ADHD and difficulties in learning. May cause headaches and migraine. Approved in the United States, European Union, New Zealand and Australia. Avoid

| 224 Avoid | Potassium metabisulphite |
|-----------|--------------------------|

**Colour: Colourless free-flowing crystals**

Has a strong sulphur dioxide odour. Protects food from oxidation and deterioration caused by micro-organisms. Used as a lemon juice preservative, as a bleaching agent for coconut cream, in the production of pickles, preservatives, beer, soft drinks, dried fruits, juices, commercially manufactured potato products including: chips and crisps, cordials and vinegar. Used in wine making. Also used in the development of photographs and photograph fixing. Can cause fainting, dizziness or unconsciousness. Known as a problem for asthmatics. Not recommended for child consumption. Can cause behavioural problems; contribute to ADHD, skin disorders: eczema, dermatitis, itching, hives and rashes. May lead to *'birth defects, genetic damage, nerve damage, severe breathing difficulties, unconsciousness, seizures, swelling in the brain, vomiting, visual disturbances, intestinal inflammation, nausea.'[94]* and severe allergic reactions. Approved in the United States, European Union, New Zealand and Australia. **Avoid**

| 225<br>**Avoid** | Potassium sulphite<br>(also called potash of<br>sulphur) (SOP) |
|---|---|

**Colour: White odourless granular powder**
Used in the production of many beverages including beer, soft drinks, dried fruits, juices, cordials, vinegar, wine and commercially produced cooked potato products. May be used as a bleaching agent in sugar production. In the human body, it is reduced to sulphate and excreted in urine. May cause allergic reactions including hyper-sensitivity, asthma, behavioural problems and contribute to ADHD, gastrointestinal reactions including stomach cramps, headaches, migraine, skin conditions including eczema, dermatitis, itching, hives and rashes. Not recommended for consumption by children. On alert in the United States and European Union. Approved in New Zealand and Australia. **Avoid**

---

[94] http://thearticlebay.com

198

| 234 Caution or Avoid | Nisin |
|---|---|

**Colour: Light brown to cream powder**
Used to extend shelf life in meats, canned fruits, beer, creams, processed cheeses also found in tomato paste. Can be a genetically engineered antibacterial peptide using the bacterium lactococcus. Not currently allowed in organic food production. Not recommended for children's consumption. Can be a problem for asthmatics or aspirin sensitive people, may irritate skin and eyes. Approved in the United States, European Union, New Zealand and Australia. **Caution** or **Avoid**

| 235 Caution | Natamycin |
|---|---|

**Colour: White to yellowish crystalline powder**
Used as a food preservative to inhibit deterioration caused by micro-organisms. Used in meats, sausages and cheeses. Can cause nausea, vomiting, anorexia, diarrhoea and skin irritation. Animal studies revealed still born. Approved in the United States, European Union, New Zealand and Australia. **Caution**

| 242 Avoid | Dimethyl dicarbonate DMDC |
|---|---|

**Colour: Colourless liquid**
Is a dangerous toxic, synthetic yeast inhibitor used in many beverages including children's juices. Used in carbonated and non-carbonated drinks, iced teas, isotonic

sports beverages, flavoured waters. As a replacement of sulphur dioxide, used in wine. If inhaled, can cause breathing difficulties, irritation to the nose, throat and respiratory tract. Can cause irritation and swelling to the skin and eyes. Has caused death. Causes cancer. *'Not recommended for consumption by children.'*[95] A re-evaluation needs to be conducted on this additive – should be banned. Approved in the United States and the European Union. On alert in New Zealand and Australia. **Avoid**

| 243 **Avoid** | Ethyl lauroyl arginate |
|---|---|

**Colour: White solid product**
Is the main compound found in coconut oil. It may be safe in small quantities, but in concentrated forms can be dangerous. Used as a food additive in non-alcoholic drinks and fruit juices, toppings, prepared salads, salted fish and specified meat products. Laboratory testing has shown multiple eye and skin irritation, breathing difficulties, nausea and vomiting. On alert in the United States and in the European Union. Approved in New Zealand and Australia
**Avoid**

| 249 **Avoid** | Potassium nitrite |
|---|---|

**Colour: Slightly yellowish granules or rods**
Is the most common preservative in the worldwide meat industry. It's a synthetic preservative. Helps to protect

---

[95] http://www.wotzinurfood.com

food against micro-organisms. Used in colour fixing in meat and fish. Is also used as a curing agent in smoked meat, fish and vegetables. Can interfere with the body's ability to carry oxygen, resulting in shortness of breath, dizziness and headaches. Will contribute towards behavioural problems. In some people will upset blood pressure. Is linked to: 'birth defects, poisoning, genetic damage, methemoglobinemia[96] (blood disorder), sudden death, tumours; severe allergic reactions.'[97] Possible carcinogen. Not permitted in foods for babies and young children. Pregnant women should avoid foods containing this preservative. Approved in the United States, European Union, New Zealand and Australia. **Avoid**

| 250 **Avoid** | Sodium nitrite |
|---|---|

**Colour: White and slightly yellowish crystals**
Is a dangerous chemical. Is used to preserve and cure meat such as ham, bacon, frankfurters and root vegetables. Prior to treatment, preserved meat can be greyish in colour; treatment allows the food to retain its pinkish colour. Studies have shown a link between Alzheimer's disease, diabetes mellitus, stomach cancer and Parkinson's disease. Other effects: blood loses its ability to carry oxygen. Symptoms: irritability, vomiting, loss of energy, headaches, difficulty in breathing, discolouration around the eyes, mouth and lips. The World Health Organisation (WHO) found that 'eating 50 grams of processed meat daily increased the risk colorectal cancer by 18 percent.'[98] Severe cases of excess sodium nitrite cause brain damage and death through suffocation due to

---

[96] An overall disability of red blood cells to release oxygen to the tissues.
[97] http://thearticlebay.com
[98] https://www.cancer.org

lack of oxygen in the lungs. Not recommended for young children and babies. Banned in Germany, Norway, Canada and Sweden. Approved in the United States, European Union, New Zealand and Australia. **Avoid**

| 251 **Avoid** | Sodium nitrate Chile saltpetre |
|---|---|

**Colour: White solid**
Known as Chilean saltpetre is a mined mineral product from the Atacama desert. Is used in the curing of meats, fish and vegetables in pickled products. Can cause asthma, gastrointestinal conditions, headaches, migraines. May also contribute to learning difficulties, behavioural problems, hyperactivity and ADHD. Can cause dizziness and asthma. Is linked to: '*birth defects, poisoning, genetic damage, methemoglobinemia (blood disorder), sudden death, tumours, cancer and severe allergic reactions.*'[99] Used as a fertiliser. Recent studies have linked it to colon cancer, and the COPD form of lung disease[100]. Approved for use in the United States, European Union, New Zealand and Australia. **Avoid**

| 252 **Avoid** | Potassium nitrate |
|---|---|

**Colour: Transparent prisms or white granular or crystalline powder**
May be derived from waste vegetable or animal matter. Helps to protect food from deterioration. Used in meat processing of salted meats such as salami, dry-cured ham,

---

[99] http://thearticlebay.com
[100] https://www.edinformatics.com

bacon, tongue, sausages, smoked frankfurters, pressed and tinned meats, pizza, and in some Dutch cheese making. In processed meat and food it can react with haemoglobin[101]. Can contribute to asthma, gastrointestinal conditions, hyperactivity, headaches, dizziness, kidney inflammation. Possibly carcinogen. Is linked to many serious health conditions, (see 251) including: upset blood pressure, vomiting, muscular weakness, vertigo, irregular pulse and limiting oxygen within the human blood supply. Prohibited in foods for infants and young children. Not recommended for infants, young children or pregnant and lactating mothers. Used as a fertiliser and in the making of fireworks and in rocket propellant. Approved for consumption in the United States, European Union, New Zealand and Australia. **Avoid**

| 260<br>**Caution** or **Avoid** | **Acetic acid glacial** |
|---|---|

**Colour: Clear and transparent liquid**
Is a synthetic product produced from wood fibres. Is used as a preservative, flavour enhancer and acidity regulator in food and food production. Used in pickles, chutneys and sauces. Is hazardous for people who suffer from any form of kidney or liver damage. May cause intestinal disorders. Can cause asthma and allergic reactions. Approved in the United States, European Union, New Zealand and Australia. **Caution** or **Avoid**

---

[101] Iron containing oxygen which allows the transporting of metalloprotein in the red bloods cells in mammals.

| 261 Caution or Avoid | Potassium acetate or potassium diacetate (i) (ii) |
|---|---|

**Colour: Clear crystals or white crystalline powder**
Is a food acidity regulator. A natural acid found in most fruits. Used in fermentation of pickles and vinegars. Also used in bouillon's, preservative in liquorice and to enhance meat and poultry flavours. Should be avoided by people with kidney disorders and disease or those with an intolerance to vinegar-based products. Will aggravate food intolerances. Contributes to headaches, intestinal upset and skin disorders. Is used in the fabric industry for the conditioning of fabric. Approved for use in the United States, European Union, New Zealand and Australia. **Caution** or **Avoid**

| 262 Caution or Avoid | Sodium acetate Sodium diacetate (i) (ii) |
|---|---|

**Colour: White odourless hygroscopic powder also granular crystals**
Acidity regulator and preservative. May be synthesised. Is used as a mould inhibitor in snack foods. Often gives potato chips their salt and vinegar flavour. Also used as a flavour enhancer in breads, cheeses, cakes and snacks. Can contribute to headaches, intestinal upset, skin disorders and severe allergic reactions. Approved in the United States. On alert in the European Union (ii). Approved in New Zealand and Australia. **Caution** or **Avoid**

| 263<br>**Caution** or **Avoid** | Calcium acetate |
|---|---|

**Colour: White crystalline solid**

Acid regulator and stabilizer; is a by-product in the manufacture of wood alcohol. Used as a thickening agent in cake mixes, puddings, pie fillings and desserts. Known to have caused mutations in animals in laboratory testing. May cause allergies and adverse reactions. Can cause nausea, vomiting, chest and abdominal pain in some people. Can contribute to birth defects and severe allergies. Approved in the United States, European Union, New Zealand and Australia. **Caution** or **Avoid**

| 270<br>**Caution** or **Avoid** | Lactic acid |
|---|---|

**Colour: Yellowish syrup**

Is the most common ingredient of fermented milk products. May be modified through biotechnical techniques. Is used in cheese and buttermilk. Also used in jams, soft margarine, cereals, marmalade, pickled red cabbage, also used in brewing beer, carbonated drinks, in manufactured sweets, (lollies) confectionary, infant milk and cereals, baby foods, pickles, mackerel, pears, sardines, salad dressings, tartare sauce and products made from strawberries and tomatoes. '*Not suitable for children and adults who are lactose intolerant. Not suitable for babies and young children; they may have difficulty in metabolising the product.*'[102] Approved in the United States, European Union, New Zealand and Australia. **Caution** or **Avoid**

---

[102] https://noshly.com

| 280 Avoid | Propionic acid |
|---|---|

**Colour: Oily, sometimes clear liquid, producing a smell resembling body odour**
Can be commercially derived from carbon monoxide, ethylene or from fermented wood pulp, natural gas and bacterial decomposing fibre. Inhibits the growth of some bacteria and mould in breads and dough products. Is linked to behavioural problems, headaches, asthma, migraine, eczema and cancer. Can cause severe allergic reactions including skin and eye irritation, choking and shortness of breath. Approved in the United States, European Union, New Zealand and Australia. **Avoid**

| 281 Avoid | Sodium propionate |
|---|---|

**Colour: White slightly yellowish compound**
Is a synthetic preservative and may be derived from ethylene and carbon monoxide or propionaldehyde or natural gas or fermented wood pulp. Is used as an antimicrobial agent preventing bacteria forming in bread. Acts as a mould inhibitor in flour. Found in processed cheese, chocolate, flour, and bread. Is thought to be linked to migraines, skin and eye irritation also behavioural problems, ADHD, learning difficulties, skill disorders and sleep disturbance. May be linked to cancer. Severe allergic reactions. Can cause shortness in breath. Can also cause flatulence nausea and abdominal discomfort. This may be a hidden food ingredient in Australia, United Kingdom and the United States. May appear as 'cultured wheat' or similar on the ingredient panel of the product. Approved in the United States, European Union, New Zealand and Australia. **Avoid**

| 282 | Calcium propionate |
|:---:|:---|
| **Avoid** | |

**Colour: White crystalline granules or powder**
Is a dangerous synthetic preservative. Is used as an antimicrobial in many food products including breads, dough, biscuits and dairy. Calcium propionate can occur naturally in small amounts in dairy produce and cheeses. The product has not been fully tested for harmful health outcomes. Eating small quantities may not be harmful but like so many additives, accumulation in the human system can take place. Has been linked to ADHD in children. Misleading diagnosis of ADHD may be due to the reaction from 282. Bowel irritability and discomfort. Can cause symptoms resembling a gall bladder attack resembling gall stones. Can also cause migraine, cancer, severe allergic reactions. Approved in the United States, European Union, New Zealand and Australia. **Avoid**

| 283 | Potassium propionate |
|:---:|:---|
| **Avoid** | |

**Colour: White colourless crystal**
Is a synthetic, dangerous, microbial preservative used in bread, bakery and dough products; is also used in pastries and dairy food. Used more widely in biscuits, cakes, buns and in many store-baked produce. Has been linked to ADHD. Misleading diagnosis of ADHD may be due to the reaction from 283. Other reactions may include migraine, gastro-intestinal upset, irritable bowel syndrome, bed wetting, eczema, nose or nasal congestion, itchy skin and rashes. On alert in the United States. Approved in the European Union, New Zealand and Australia. **Avoid**

| 290 Caution or Avoid | Carbon dioxide |
|---|---|

**Colour: Colourless, odourless gas**

An acidity regulator derived from lime manufacture is also a propellant[103]. Used in fizzy alcoholic and soft drinks, sparkling wine, fruit juice and confectionary. Also used in fire extinguishers. Possible links to *'impaired infertility',* *neurotoxicity'*[104] and stomach ulcers. Approved in the United States, European Union, New Zealand and Australia. Caution or Avoid

| 296 Caution or Avoid | Malic acid |
|---|---|

**Colour: White crystalline powder**

L malic acid is a naturally occurring organic acid that is found in many fruits and vegetables. Used as an acidity regulator. Commercial malic acid is a synthetic substance derived from heated, under pressure, malic acid and sulphuric acid. Used in food and drink products to inhibit bacteria. Also used in jams, liqueur making, candy and confectionary. Can be found in some health drinks. It can help to limit natural fatigue. Is linked to eczema. Can contribute to mouth, throat or stomach irritation, contribute to bloating and gas, diarrhoea, acid reflux and upset stomach. Not recommended for children and infants. Approved in the United States, European Union, New Zealand and Australia. Caution or Avoid

---

[103] A propellant is a chemical substance used in the development of energy or pressured gas.
[104] http://thearticlebay.com

| 297 **Caution** | Fumaric acid |
|---|---|

**Colour: Odourless white crystalline powder**

Used as an acidity regulator. Is found in plants of the genus Fumaria. Used as an antioxidant or raising agent in breads, cake mixes and soft drinks. Linked to eczema. People may have adverse reactions if suffering with allergies or food reactions. Approved in the United States, European Union, New Zealand and Australia **Caution**

**Your Notes**

........................................................................
........................................................................
........................................................................
........................................................................
........................................................................
........................................................................
........................................................................
........................................................................
........................................................................
........................................................................
........................................................................
........................................................................
........................................................................
........................................................................
........................................................................
........................................................................
........................................................................
........................................................................
........................................................................
........................................................................

# Devils: Antioxidants (300 range)

| Devil Numbers | Additive |
|:---:|:---:|
| 300 **Caution** | Ascorbic acid Vitamin C |

**Colour: Slightly yellowish crystalline powder**
Naturally occurs in fresh fruit and vegetables. Can be synthetically made from genetically modified corn (maize) for the mass food market. In some foods, used as an anti-oxidant. Added to breakfast cereal, frozen fish, wine, concentrated milk products, flour, meat and cured meats and tinned baby foods. Overdoses can result in kidney stones, vomiting, diarrhoea and dizziness. May encourage arthritic conditions. Read the label when buying baby food. Approved in the European Union, United States, New Zealand and Australia. **Caution**

| Devil Numbers | Additive |
|:---:|:---:|
| 301 **Avoid** | Sodium ascorbate |

**Colour: White or almost white, odourless crystalline powder**
Is used as an antioxidant in bread and cooked food. May be derived from genetically modified corn (maize). Is a synthetic substance. Can cause adverse effects which include difficulties in breathing, rashes on skin, itching, hives, tightness in the chest, swelling of the mouth, lips, tongue or face. Muscle weakness, severe diarrhoea and carcinogens. Approved in the United States, European Union, New Zealand and Australia. **Avoid**

| 302 | Calcium ascorbate |
| Safe or Caution | |

**Colour: Light yellow crystalline powder**
Vitamin C occurs naturally in fruit and vegetables. Vitamin C is essential for growth, healthy teeth, bones and blood vessels. It helps in the absorption of iron. Is used as an antioxidant, colour preservative and vitamin supplement. Synthesized calcium ascorbate is used in scotch eggs, bouillons and other food products. May increase the development of kidney stones. Approved for use in the United States, European Union, New Zealand and Australia. Safe or Caution

| 303 | Potassium ascorbate |
| Caution or Avoid | |

**Colour: White odourless crystalline powder**
Used as an antioxidant in food and in vitamin C. Maybe safe in some instances. Used in dairy-based drinks, processed cheese, fat-based cheeses, breakfast cereals, canned or bottled vegetables, egg-based desserts, pasta, batters, vinegars, mustards, and vinegar-based condiments. Overuse may lead to diarrhoea, mood swings, rashes, itching, difficulty in breathing, swelling of the mouth, face, lips and tongue, weakness and bone pain. Not permitted as a food additive in the United Kingdom, the European Union and the United States. Approved in New Zealand and Australia. Caution or Avoid

| 304 **Safe** | Ascorbyl palmitate |
|---|---|

**Colour: White or yellowish-white solid**

Is a combination of fatty acid palmitate combined with ascorbic acid. Does naturally occur in most fruit and vegetables. Is plant extracted and prevents food from oxidation. Acts as a preservative. Approved in the United States, European Union, New Zealand and Australia. **Safe**

| 307 **Caution** | α-Tocopherol or vitamin E |
|---|---|

**Colour: Is a class of chemical compounds**

A synthetic vitamin E antioxidant. Found in genetically modified plants such as maize, soy and cotton. Natural vitamin E is found in natural oils: eggs and leafy vegetables. Also found in vegetable oils such as: wheat germ, soy, rice germ, cottonseed and maize. Works as an antioxidant for fatty acids and tissue fats preventing vitamin A from oxidation. Used in margarine and salad dressings. The natural Mediterranean diet is rich in natural vitamin E. Recent studies suggest it may help with the reduction of heart disease and cancer. On alert in the United States, European Union, New Zealand and Australia. **Caution**

| 307b **Caution** | Tocopherols concentrate, mixed |
|---|---|

**Colour: Brown to red viscous oil**
Synthetic vitamin E. '*Is produced from genetically altered (GMO) crops such as soybeans or corn. Used extensively in vitamins sold in regular stores and health food stores.*'[105] On alert in the United States. Approved in the European Union, New Zealand and Australia**. Caution**

| 308 **Caution** | α-Tocopherol - synthetic |
|---|---|

**As 307, 307b above**

| 309 **Caution** | γ-Tocopherol. - synthetic |
|---|---|

**As 307, 307b and 308 above**

---

[105] http://thearticlebay.com

| 310 **Avoid** | Propyl gallate |
|---|---|

**Colour: White to cream crystalline solid**

Is synthesised and a by-product of plant tannins. Also produced from nut galls.[106] Used in some restricted food groups. Used in lard, margarine, salad dressing, oils and some packaging. Protects foods from deterioration caused by oxidation. Causes allergic reactions, asthma, gastrointestinal discomfort and associated health conditions, skin disorders including: eczema, dermatitis, itching, hives and rashes. May cause blood disorders. Linked to cancer. Asthmatics and those sensitive to aspirin should avoid. Is linked to reproductive difficulties and prevents the absorption of iron. People with liver or kidney conditions avoid. Not suitable for babies and young children. May cause hyperactivity. Approved in the United States, European Union, New Zealand and Australia. **Avoid**

| 311 **Caution** or **Avoid** | Octyl gallate |
|---|---|

**Colour: Cream to white crystalline solid**

Derived from nut galls. Is used as an antioxidant and found in dairy foods, margarine, edible fat, oils, reduced fat spread and salad oils. Asthmatics and aspirin sensitive people should avoid. May cause skin irritation such as urticaria. In some instances, may cause gastric irritation and stomach upset. Can also cause hyperactivity and insomnia. Not suitable for babies or small children. Feeding mothers

---

[106] An abnormal outgrowth of plant tissue which resembles a nut, but should not be mistaken for a nut. Used in many additives.

should avoid. Approved in the United States, European Union, New Zealand and Australia. Caution or Avoid

| 315 Caution | Erythorbic acid |
|---|---|

**Colour: A crystalline compound**
A vegetable-based derivative from sucrose or genetically modified corn (maize). Is a synthetic antioxidant. Used in dairy-based drinks, cheeses, breakfast cereals, fat-based spreads, canned vegetables, processed fruit, vinegar, mustards and sweeteners. No known side effects to date. Approved in the United States, European Union, New Zealand and Australia. Caution

| 316 Caution or Avoid | Sodium erythorbate |
|---|---|

**Colour: Almost white crystalline powder**
Is a synthetic antioxidant. Can be genetically modified from corn (maize). Is used in meat and poultry to prevent bacillus cereus from developing. Also used in hot dogs and beef sticks, curing of ham, in a variety of cheeses, canned and dried vegetables and as an antioxidant and bread improver. Added to the ingredients in soft drinks. Possible short-term side effects: headaches, body flushes, fatigue, dizziness and hemolysis.[107] Long-term effects could be kidney stones and gout. Could cause irritation to skin and eyes. On alert in the United States. Approved in the European Union, New Zealand and Australia. Caution or Avoid

---

[107] The rupturing of red blood cells and the release of their contents into surrounding fluid.

| 319 Avoid | tert-Butylhydroquinone (TBHQ) |
|---|---|

**Colour: Light or white mahogany crystal**
Derived from petroleum is highly toxic and a dangerous synthetic used as an antioxidant in many foods. TBHQ is a form of butane used in oils as an anti-foaming agent and in Silly Putty.[108] Is used in edible oils, margarines and fats, drippings, salad dressing, dried fish products, biscuits, quick cooking rice, canned nuts, noodles, cracker biscuits, snack foods, bacon products and many dairy foods. Used to extend shelf life and reduce rancidity. Also used in paint products, varnishes and skin care products. Is linked to hyperactivity in some children. Can cause depression, cancer, difficulty in concentration and sleep deprivation, nausea, tantrums, tinnitus (ringing in the ears), dizziness and a sense of suffocation. Dangerous for asthmatics. May cause vomiting and delirium. Can affect cholesterol levels and have severe allergic reactions. A dose of 5g is considered fatal. Not suitable for babies and young children, pregnant or lactating mothers. In animal studies, TBHQ was identified in the impairment of T cell response to the flu virus.[109] On alert in the United States. Approved in the European Union, New Zealand and Australia. **Avoid**

| 320 Avoid | Butylated hydroxyanisole (BHA) |
|---|---|

**Colour: White or slightly yellow, waxy crystals**
Derived from petroleum, again highly toxic and banned in Japan since 1958. Is a synthetic version of vitamin E. Is used in the manufacture of chewing gum, instant potato

---

[108] A toy based on silicone polymers.
[109] http://www.sci-news.com

products, fried snacks, margarine, edible oils, fats, fat products, soft drinks, nuts, cereals, biscuits, cakes, pastry, pastry products, sweets, lollies and confectionary. Found in some sauces. Not permitted in infant foods. Concerns over carcinogenicity and estrogenic effects. May cause hyperactivity, asthma and adverse breathing reactions, allergies and insomnia. Is linked to: *'liver damage, lung-stomach and ovarian tumours, is stored in body tissue, chronic urticaria, conjunctivitis, headaches, skin blisters, throat and chest pain, increases behavioural changes, reproductive difficulties, birth defects, dermatitis and changes in blood values.'*[110] Tumours found in animal research. Not recommended for babies and young children. Has been linked to cancer. Banned in some countries. Due to pressure from the food industry, not banned in the United Kingdom. On alert in the United States. Approved in the European Union, New Zealand and Australia. **Avoid**

| 321 **Avoid** | Butylated hydroxytoluene |
|---|---|

**Colour: Slightly yellowish crystal**
Is a petroleum derivative and a synthetic antioxidant. Is used in the commercial and mass production of food. Used in commercially manufactured biscuits, cakes, fats, oils, sweets, lollies, confectionary, cereals, including breakfast cereals, edible oils, oil products, nuts and nut products, fats, margarine, pastry and pastry products, ice cream, lard, fat, cheese spreads and potato products. Also used in many medicines. Can cause insomnia, skin rashes, urticaria, problems with liver metabolism and reproductive failures. Causes hyperactivity, behavioural problems, learning difficulties, asthma and skin conditions, including: eczema, dermatitis, hives and skin problems. Not permitted in infant and children's food. Should be avoided

---

[110] http://thearticlebay.com

by feeding and lactating mothers. Possible links to cell division. Banned in Japan. Due to industry pressure, this antioxidant is still used in the United Kingdom. Banned in some countries. The European Union has restricted the use of this chemical. Approved in New Zealand and Australia. **Avoid**

| 322 Safe or Caution | Lecithin also Lecithin (i) (ii) |
|---|---|

**Colour: Yellowish-brown fatty substance**
Is used as a food additive, emulsifier, antioxidant, flavour protector, thickener and gelling agent. Is a commercially synthetic substance derived from lecithin, soya, which may be genetically modified (GM), and the main source of lecithin, including egg yolks, peanuts, legume seed, rape seed, sunflowers, maize and animal sources. Methods of extraction should always be considered when buying this product. In commercially, synthetically derived lecithin, hexane and acetone, (both dangerous solvents), are used to extract lecithin from its source. Lecithin is within all living cells and is a component of brain and nerve cells. It protects the membranes of unsaturated fats from oxygen invasion. Synthetic Lecithin is used in margarine, it stabilises emulsions, improves textures and flavours in spreads. Is also used in dough, bakery products, it reduces fat and egg requirements and protects yeast cells. It allows for combining oils, fats and water in chocolate, margarine, ice cream and mayonnaise; is also used in some milk powders. Read the product information before purchase. Overdose may upset the stomach and cause profuse sweating. Approved in the United States, European Union, New Zealand and Australia. **Safe** or **Caution**

**Your Notes**

.............................................................................
.............................................................................
.............................................................................
.............................................................................
.............................................................................
.............................................................................
.............................................................................
.............................................................................
.............................................................................
.............................................................................
.............................................................................
.............................................................................
.............................................................................
.............................................................................
.............................................................................
.............................................................................
.............................................................................
.............................................................................

# Devils: More food acids (300 range)

| Devil Numbers | Additive |
|---|---|
| **325** <br> Caution or Avoid | **Sodium lactate (food acid)** |

**Colour: Colourless, odourless transparent liquid**
Is used as an acidity regulator; may contain pork rennin. Sodium lactate is not a by-product of milk. Sodium lactate is derived from non-dairy produce such as corn starch, potatoes, molasses, sugar and tapioca. Occasionally, sodium lactate may be produced from whey which then may be returned to the production of dairy produce. Used in the production of sponge cakes, Swiss rolls, cheeses, jams, jellies, margarine, sweets, lollies, confectionary, ice cream pharmaceutical preparation, the manufacturing of noodles, sea and poultry production. Also used in pre-manufactured roast food, some flavouring and as an antiseptic for meat. Side effects may include: chest pain, wheezing, muscle cramps and inability to focus. *'May cause liver disease in children.*[111] Not recommended for babies, young children and lactating mothers. Approved in the United States, European Union, New Zealand and Australia. Caution or Avoid

| **326** <br> Caution or Avoid | **Potassium lactate** |
|---|---|

**Colour: White potassium salt of lactic acid**
In food manufacture it's genetically modified and engineered. May be derived from whey, pork and may

---

[111] http://thearticlebay.com

contain rennin. Found in confectionary, cheeses, ice cream, fruit jellies, some soups and canned fruit. As 325, *'May cause liver damage in children.'* Not recommended for babies and small children as it increases the antioxidants of other substances. Children have not developed the enzymes in the liver to process these foods. Approved in the United States, European Union, New Zealand and Australia. **Caution** or **Avoid**

| 327 **Caution** | Calcium lactate |
|---|---|

**Colour: White crystalline salt**
Is an acidity regulator extracted from milk; may contain pork, rennin and whey. Is used in the food and medicinal industries. In food is used as an ingredient in baking powder. Is also used as a flour treatment agent. Also used in powdered and condensed milk. Added to tinned fruits and vegetables which react with pectin. Found in marmalades, jams and jellies. Also found in sugar-free food and chewing gum. As this additive is derived from animal sources, young children and babies with milk intolerance could show adverse reactions. Also, pregnant and feeding mothers should avoid. Approved in the European Union, United States, New Zealand and Australia. **Caution**

| 328 **Caution** or **Avoid** | Ammonium lactate |
|---|---|

**Colour: White solid or liquid**
Is used as a food additive which regulates acidity and alkalinity in commercially produced food. Is used as a treatment for flour also used in confectionary, lollies,

sweets, salad dressing, cakes, biscuits, ready to eat poultry or meat products, tinned fruit and vegetables, yogurt, wheat beers, soft drinks and infant formulas. Produced by the fermentation of lactose (milk sugar) commercially from bacterial fermentation of carbohydrates and molasses. Not safe for babies and young children. Commercially produced from lactose. People with lactose intolerance may show adverse reactions. On alert in the United States and the European Union. Approved in New Zealand and Australia. **Caution** or **Avoid**

| 329 **Caution** or **Avoid** | Magnesium lactate DL |
|---|---|

**Colour: White crystalline powder**
Is added to some foods and beverages. Acts as an acidity regulator and flour treatment agent. Is derived from milk and may contain pork rennin or whey. May cause bloating, gas, upset stomach, hives, difficulty in breathing, swelling of the face, tongue, lips and throat. Not recommended for babies, young children, feeding or lactating mothers. On alert in the United States and the European Union. Approved in New Zealand and Australia. **Caution** or **Avoid**

| 330 **Avoid** | Citric acid |
|---|---|

**Colour: White crystals**
Is an acidity regulator. May be naturally derived from citrus fruits. In commercial production citric acid always contains Process-Free Glutamic Acid or (PFGA). Please see additive 620 www.thearticlebay.com. ('*620 is a manufactured, highly refined, isolated and unbound chemical containing*

223

*L-glutamic acid and dangerous pollutants that always contain D-glutamic acid (a proven neuropoison),* or nerve poison, '*pyroglutamin acid and other harmful pollutants such as mono-and dichlopropnols* (a possible carcinogen) *which are not removable.*[112] This product is used as a preservative and flavouring to add sourness to sweets, lollies, confectionery and as a preservative in soft drinks. Is also used in biscuit and cake making, canned fish, infant formulas, cheese making, rye bread and fermented meats. In commercial production, is a genetically engineered product produced from corn. May cause problems to MSG sensitive people. Can cause tooth decay. Other serious health conditions include: arthritic symptoms, eating disorders leading to obesity, ADHD, depression and severe depression, personality disorders, schizophrenia and paranoia. Can also be found in most Asian cooking leading to a condition known as Chinese Restaurant Syndrome (CRS). Approved in the United States, European Union, New Zealand and Australia. **Avoid**

| 331 **Avoid** | Sodium citrates: **(i) Sodium dihydrogen citrate (ii) Disodium monohydrogen citrate (iii) Trisodium citrate** |
|---|---|

**Colour: Colourless or white crystalline powder or granule**
Are sodium salts of citric acid found as a compound in every living cell. Large concentrations are found in strawberries, citrus fruit and other fruit. For mass-market consumption it is commercially synthesized from sugar beet, corn-based starch and molasses which are mainly genetically modified crops. Used as a food regulator to increase aroma and strength in marmalades, jams or conserves. Also used in gelatine products including: ice

---

[112] http://thearticlebay.com

cream, carbonated drinks, evaporated and condensed milk, wine, tinned vegetables, milk powder and processed cheese. It also decreases browning in fruit products. May lead to headaches, intestinal upset and constipation. Please see 330, Citric acid and the related information of 620, Processes-Free Glutamic Acid (PFGA). A dangerous food additive. Approved in the United States, European Union, New Zealand and Australia. **Avoid**

| 332 **Caution** or **Avoid** | Potassium citrate and Potassium dihydrogen citrate (i) Tripotassium citrate (ii) |
|---|---|

**Colour: Transparent crystals or white powder**
Is an acidity regulator which is derived from genetically modified crops. Please see 330 Citric acid and the related information of 620 (PFGA). Is used in soft drinks and lite lemonade products and drinks. Used as an alkanizing agent in treatments of urinary tract infections and cystitis. Used in the reduction of kidney stones. Before use, seek medical advice if there are kidney problems. On alert in the United States and in the European Union: potassium citrates. Approved in New Zealand and Australia. On alert in the United States and the European Union, Potassium dihydrogen citrate (i). Approved in New Zealand and Australia. On alert in the United States and European Union Tripotassium citrate (ii). Approved in New Zealand and Australia. **Caution** or **Avoid**

| 333 **Caution** or **Avoid** | Calcium citrate Monosodium citrate (i) Dicalcium citrate (ii) Tricalcium citrate (iii) |
|---|---|

**Colour: Needle shaped crystals**
Can occur naturally in citrus fruits. For commercial and mass-market production is synthesised and used as a food

acidity regulator, food preservative, food additive, antioxidant, flavour enhancer and firming agent. Used in gelatine products including ice cream, carbonated drinks and beverages, wine, jams, evaporated and condensed milk, preserves, tinned vegetables, milk powders and processed cheeses. Can cause mouth ulcers, allergies or adverse reactions. May contribute to arthritic symptoms. Commercial Citric acid is developed through gene modifications where micro-organisms grown on culture media that usually contains glucose, molasses (sugar beet) or maize starch. Maize starch is derived from genetically modified maize. High consumption of potassium can rupture blood cells, add to tissue and liver damage and lead to arrhythmia which can lead to cardiac arrest. All 333 additives are on alert in the United States, in the European Union, New Zealand and Australia. **Caution** or **Avoid**

| 334<br>**Caution** or **Avoid** | Tartaric acid |
|---|---|

**Colour: White crystalline organic acid**
Found as a natural ingredient in unripened fruit including: grapes, bananas, tamarinds and citrus. Is synthesised as a by-product during and after wine making. Is used in baking powder, jelly, tinned fruit and vegetables, cocoa powder, chewing gum, frozen dairy produce, beverages, dried egg whites, bakery products, jams, preserves, tinned tomatoes, asparagus and tomatoes. Is used as a fertiliser, for cleaning surfaces of copper, aluminium, iron and alloys. Can cause allergies and adverse reactions. Also headaches, damage to intestinal microbiota and constipation. Approved in the United States, European Union, New Zealand and Australia. **Caution** or **Avoid**

| 335<br>Caution or Avoid | Sodium tartrate<br>(i) Monosodium tartrate<br>(ii)Disodium tartrate |
|---|---|

**Colour: Colourless crystal or white crystalline powder**

Is commercially synthesised and a by-product of the wine industry. Is used as a food acidity regulator, binding agent and antioxidant. Used in jellies, baking powder, chewing gum, sweets, tinned fruits and vegetables, cocoa powder, margarine, carbonated drinks, frozen dairy products and sausages. Those people with heart or kidney conditions should avoid. May contribute to headaches, damage to the intestinal microbiota and contribute to constipation. Inhalation can contribute to breathing difficulties, stomach cramps and dizziness. 335 approved in the United States, European Union, New Zealand and Australia. 335 (i) and (ii) on alert in the United States, European Union, New Zealand and Australia. Caution or Avoid

| 336<br>Caution or Avoid | Potassium tartrates or<br>Potassium acid tartrates<br>(i) Monopotassium<br>tartrate<br>(ii) Dipotassium tartrate |
|---|---|

**Colour: White crystalline powder**

Used as an acid regulator and food stabiliser. Found in most food products including sweets, lollies, confectionary, jams and carbonated drinks. Will exacerbate headaches, damage to intestinal microbiota, aggravate intestinal upset and encourage constipation. Can lead to damaged or impaired liver and kidney problems, high blood pressure and heart problems. On alert in the United States, European Union, New Zealand and Australia. Caution or Avoid

| 337 Caution or Avoid | Sodium potassium tartrates |
|---|---|

**Colour: Colourless crystals or as a white crystalline powder**

Is an antioxidant, acid regulator, stabiliser and mineral salt found in most commercially manufactured foods. These include: meat, pasteurised and processed chesses, jams and margarines. Is used in cola drinks to offset intense sweetness. Disodium hydrogen phosphate is added to milk powder to prevent sticking or lumping. May cause headaches, damage to intestinal microbiota, intestinal upset and constipation. Also allergies or adverse reactions. People with kidney or heart conditions should avoid. Can lead to absorbent and brittle bones leading to osteoporosis. Is dangerous for people with high blood pressure, damaged or impaired liver function and heart problems. Is also used as a laxative. Banned in organic foods. Also used in textile dyeing. On alert in the United States. Approved in the European Union, New Zealand and Australia. Caution or Avoid

| 338 Avoid | Phosphoric acid |
|---|---|

**Colour: Transparent syrup**

Derived from phosphate ore. Is an acidity regulator and added to foods; is also used as a preservative. Used in many cola and like drinks also other soda fizzy drinks, cereal bars, processed meats, bottled coffee and beverages, some cheeses and pickled products. Is also used as a phosphate in fertilizers, agricultural feed, soaps, polishes, waxes and detergents. Other uses: the coagulation of rubber latex, soil re-stabilization, as a catalyst for the production of propylene and butane polymers. Also used as a rust protector in the car and electrical industries. Can lead to digestive disorders and links between kidney disease, kidney stones and osteoporosis. Has a negative effect on the body's nervous system and can cause damage to intestinal and microbiota. Continuous exposure may cause bronchitis, phlegm, shortness of breath, drying and cracking of skin. May be linked to cardiovascular disease. Approved in the United States, European Union, New Zealand and Australia. **Avoid**

**Your Notes**

...............................................................................

...............................................................................

...............................................................................

...............................................................................

...............................................................................

...............................................................................

...............................................................................

...............................................................................

...............................................................................

...............................................................................

...............................................................................

...............................................................................

...............................................................................

...............................................................................

...............................................................................

...............................................................................

...............................................................................

...............................................................................

...............................................................................

...............................................................................

# Devils: Mineral salts (300 range)

| Devil Numbers | Additive |
|:---:|:---:|
| 339<br>Avoid | Sodium phosphates<br>(i) Sodium dihydrogen phosphate<br>(ii) Disodium hydrogen phosphate<br>(iii) Trisodium phosphate |

**Colour: White granular or crystalline solid**
Sodium phosphates are part of the cell makeup of the human body. Additive produced in Europe from animal bones and in the United States mined from phosphate. May be synthetic. Is commercially produced and used in condensed milk for coagulation. Used as an anti-caking agent in desserts and puddings. Added to some cereal products to brighten the colour. Used in cheeses to help keep their shape and melting properties. Also added to bread, cakes and baked goods, cola drinks and used in laxative preparation. Used to off-set extreme sweetness in commercially produced food products. Kidneys excrete the substance by bonding with calcium taken from the bones in the human body which leaves them brittle and porous with an increase to osteoporosis. Is linked to kidney stones. May contribute to digestive disorders, skin conditions including: eczema, dermatitis, itching and hives. High intakes may upset the body's calcium phosphorous balance. Is banned in organic food. Other products using this additive include: toilet cleaners, stain removers, dishwashing detergent, industrial solvents, mildew remover, lead abating agents to clean exterior walls before painting. Also used as a fixing agent in textile dyeing. Approved in the United States, European Union, New Zealand and Australia 339 and 339 (i). On alert in the United States, European Union, New Zealand and Australia 339 (ii) (iii). Avoid

| 340<br>**Avoid** | **Potassium phosphate, dibasic**<br>(i) Potassium dihydrogen phosphate<br>(ii)Dipotassium hydrogen phosphate<br>(iii) Tripotassium phosphate |
|---|---|

**Colour: White crystalline powder**

Naturally occurs, in small quantities in the body. For commercial use is mined in the United States. Phosphates from Europe are acquired from animal bones. In food, used as an acidity regulator, chelating agent, antioxidant which protects food from deterioration, and stabiliser. Used in jellies and jelly products, cooked and cured meats, drinking chocolate, milk and cream powders and their products. High intake can lead to tissue and kidney damage, the rupture of blood cells, heart arrhythmia and cardiac arrest. Can bind up the body's calcium supply and is linked to kidney stones. 340 approved in the United States, European Union, New Zealand and Australia. On alert in the United States and the European Union, (i), (ii) and (iii). Approved in New Zealand and Australia 340 (ii) and (iii). **Avoid**

| 341<br>**Caution** or **Avoid** | **Calcium phosphate**<br>(i) Calcium dihydrogen phosphate<br>(ii) Calcium hydrogen phosphate<br>(iii)Tricalcium phosphate |
|---|---|

**Colour: White powder**

Is used as an anti-caking agent and an acidity regulator in baking powder. Also used as a bread enhancer and enhancer in bakery products in commercial bread and bakery production. Is used in spices as an anti-caking agent. Also used as a food regulator, anti-caking agent, firming agent and humectant. In Europe is extracted from animal bones. In the United States is produced from phosphorous mined phosphates. May be used as a dietary supplement in prepared breakfast cereals, enriched flour, noodle products, baking powder, cake mixes, doughnuts and muffins. Used in the pharmaceutical industry in tablet preparation and as a body odour deterrent. High levels of calcium phosphates lead to digestive disorders, tissue damage and rupture of blood cells also damage to the kidneys and heart. May contribute to arrhythmia which may lead to cardiac arrest. Used as a polishing agent in enamels. Approved in the United States. On alert in the European Union (i), (ii). Approved in New Zealand and Australia. **Caution** or **Avoid**

| 342<br>**Avoid**<br> | **Ammonium phosphates**<br>**(i) Ammonium dihydrogen phosphate**<br>**(ii) Diammonium hydrogen phosphate** |
|---|---|

**Colour: White to clear crystal**

In small quantities naturally occurs in fruit and vegetables. In commercial production, ammonium phosphates are the salts produced from ammonium rock and sulphur. Ammonia is used to help dissolve rock. Is also used as an acidity regulator and firming agent and to maintain food strength. Is used in flour production to maintain baking quality and flour colour. Used as a yeast nutrient in some wine and mead making. Used in some brands of cigarettes and in the purification of sugar. Also used in the production of fertilisers and animal feed. If handling, may cause skin and eye irritation. Approved in the United States: Diammonium hydrogen phosphate (ii). On alert ammonium phosphates and Ammonium phosphate (i). On alert in the European Union Ammonium phosphate (i) and (ii). All approved in New Zealand and Australia. **Avoid**

| 343<br>Caution | Magnesium phosphate<br>(i) Magnesium dihydrogen phosphate<br>(ii) Magnesium hydrogen phosphate<br>(iii) Trimagnesium phosphate |
|---|---|

**Colour: Odourless white crystalline powder**

A natural mineral salt that is found in whole grains, legumes, broccoli, squash, dairy products and almonds. Magnesium is part of our chemistry which is found in the body including: brain, heart, spinal cord, liver, lungs, pancreas, spleen, kidneys, thyroid gland, intestines and in nerve and muscle cells. Commercially available in Europe which is obtained from animal bones. In the United States is obtained from minerals. Is used as an acidity regulator and anti-caking agent in the bakery and food industries also used in food supplements which increases the activity of antioxidants. If supplementing your diet, seek professional advice. May have several side effects when used as a dietary supplement. In larger than prescribed quantities may cause vomiting, abdominal cramps, may irritate the intestinal tract. Magnesium is absorbed in the small intestine and excreted via the kidneys. Excessive magnesium may lead to tissue damage, ruptured blood cells, kidney damage and heart arrhythmia that can lead to cardiac arrest. Approved in the United States, European Union, New Zealand and Australia. Caution

| 349 **Avoid** | Ammonium malate |
|---|---|

**Colour: Colourless white crystalline powder**
Is the ammonium[113] salt of malic acid. As a manufactured additive is used in the food industry as a flour treatment, firming agent and acidity regulator. Is used in flour as a buffer agent in confectionary, soft drinks and other foods and drinks. Manufacturers use it to prolong shelf life in the production of processed foods for the mass and commercial food market. Very little information available. Is used as a fertiliser. On alert in the United States and in the European Union. Approved in New Zealand and Australia. **Avoid**

| 350 **Avoid** | Sodium hydrogen malate<br>**(i) Sodium hydrogen DL – malate**<br>**(ii) Sodium DL malate** |
|---|---|

**Colour: Odourless white powder**
Used in sweetened coconut. Low salt substitute. A natural acid present in fruit. Is an acidity regulator and flavouring agent. Used in a range of fruit drinks, soft drinks and dairy blends. Possibly harmful for the human brain and nervous systems. More research is needed on this additive. On alert in the United States, European Union, New Zealand and Australia. **Avoid**

---

[113] A possible threat to the environment. Used in soldering flux as a fertiliser and many other uses. It doesn't belong in food.

| 351 Caution | Potassium malates (i) Potassium hydrogen malate (ii) Potassium malate |
|---|---|

**Colour: Colourless crystalline powder**

Is a natural acid found in fruit. Commercially produced by combining two types of synthesised product including: (i) potassium hydrogen malate, and (ii) potassium malate. Is used as an acidifier and food regulator. Used in canned vegetables, soft drinks, fruit products, soups and sauces. Also used in low-salt substitute products, and in many commercially produced fruit drinks, sweetened coconut, soft drinks including fruit squash, dairy blend products, tinned pulses, tinned tomatoes, tinned fruit and vegetables, jams, preserves, potato snacks, sweets, lollies, confectionary, spaghetti sauce, frozen vegetables, jelly and jelly products. Not allowed in infant food as they do not have the necessary gut enzymes to metabolise synthetic additives. All malates on alert in the United States. Potassium malates and potassium malate (ii) approved in the European Union New Zealand and Australia. **Caution**

| 352 Safe or Caution | Calcium malate (i) Calcium hydrogen malate (ii) Calcium malate, D, L- |
|---|---|

**Colour: White mineral salt of malic acid**

Is used as a food additive. May be used as a dietary supplement. Used as a thickener and flavouring. May be synthetic. Can be found in ice cream, fried products, marmalades, sweetened coconut, most fruit drinks, fruit squash, low-salt substitute foods, dairy blend foods, jams and conserves, potato snacks, frozen vegetables, tinned tomatoes, jelly and jelly products, sweets, lollies and confectionary and spaghetti sauces. If synthetic, not allowed in infant food as they do not have the necessary enzymes to metabolise imitation additives. On alert in the United States. Approved in the European Union, New Zealand and Australia. Safe or Caution

| 353 Caution | Metatartaric acid |
|---|---|

**Colour: White slightly yellowish crystalline organic acid**
Is a by-product of the wine industry and is added to wine to reduce surplus acid used in fruit juices. Metabolises to tartaric acid in the human body. Eighty percent is destroyed by bacteria in the intestines. Mostly safe but not allowed in infant or young children's food as they do not have the enzyme capacity to metabolise these compounds. On alert in the United States. Approved in the European Union, New Zealand and Australia. Caution

| 354 Caution or Avoid | Calcium tartrate |
|---|---|

**Colour: Pure crystalline salt of tartaric acid**
A natural acid present in fresh fruit. Is a by-product of the wine industry made from the left over pulp of wine making. The waste products, after fermentation, are neutralised by heating then treated with calcium hydroxide, then with sulphuric acid to produce tartrate acid. In the United states, calcium tartrate is made from unfermented crushed grapes. Used in fish and fruit preserves, seaweed products and as a preservative in tobacco in the United Kingdom. Found in some biscuits and baby/infant rusks. Is used as a food modifying agent in some infant foods. Not recommended for infants as they lack the necessary enzymes to metabolise these compounds. May cause

gastro-enteritis in some people. On alert in the United States. Approved in the European Union, New Zealand and Australia. **Caution** or **Avoid**

| 355 **Avoid** | Adipic acid |
|---|---|

**Colour: White crystalline**
Originally a by-product from beet or sugarcane. Is now a synthetic extracted from beetroot or nitric acid using highly toxic petroleum hexanes. Is a mineral salt. Used as a rising agent. Is used in a wide range of foods as a flavouring and jellying compound. It allows jelly-type foods to become fizzy, firm and have texture. Found in the tart flavour of gelatine and fruit juices. Used in cake mixes, pudding mixes, manufactured baked goods, ice blocks, some cheeses, dairy products, pickles, tart condiments, ice blocks and margarine. Also used in the manufacture of nylon, carpet making, automobile products and clothing. Aggravates food intolerances, including eye irritation. *'May contribute to nausea, diarrhoea and delayed growth.'*[114] On alert in the United States. Approved in the European Union, New Zealand and Australia. **Avoid**

| 357 **Avoid** | Potassium adipate |
|---|---|

**Colour: Chemical compound**
Was a natural acid present in sugar cane juice and beets. Is now commercially produced from nitric acid by extraction from beetroot using highly toxic petroleum

---

[114] http://thearticlebay.com

hexanes. Used as an acidity regulator to alter the acidity of food. Used as a gelling and firming agent in baking powder; also used in many fruit drinks, beer, jams and conserves, pudding mixes, ice blocks and flavoured ice products, margarine, and antacid medicines. Used in low-sodium herbal products. Also used in the production of PVC and plastics. Can lead to tissue damage and the rupture of blood vessels, kidney and heart damage and heart arrhythmia that can lead to cardiac arrest. May also lead to diarrhoea, delayed growth. Abnormally high levels can have fatal results. Further research is needed. On alert in the United States. Approved in the European Union, New Zealand and Australia. **Avoid**

| 359 Caution or Avoid | Ammonium adipates |
|---|---|

**Colour: Is the ammonium salt of adipic acid**
Is the ammonium salt of adipic acid and works as a food additive when used in cooking. Adipates are found in a number of different foods, including: *'fermented milks, beverage whiteners, many types of processed cheese, dairy-based desserts including: ice cream, ice milk, milk, fruit or flavoured yogurts, fats and oils, margarine, butter and margarine blends, fat-based desserts, fruit preparations, including pulp, purees, fruit topping and coconut milk, fruit-based desserts including fruit-flavoured water-based desserts, fruit fillings and pastries, vegetables and seaweeds in vinegar, oil, brine or soy sauce, vegetable and nut and seed pulps and preparation (e.g., vegetable desserts and sauces, candied vegetables, soybean curd), cooked and fried vegetables and seaweed, cocoa-based spreads, including fillings, hard and soft confectionary including nougat, chewing gum, fine bakery items, topping (non-fruit) and sweet sauces, pre-cooked or dried pastas and noodles and similar products, cereal and starch based dessert (e.g., rice and tapioca pudding), batters including:*

*fish and poultry batter, baking and baking products, processed meat, poultry, game in whole or cuts, egg-based desserts including custards, herbs, spices, seasoning including: salt substitutes and condiments and seasoning for instant noodles, soups and broths, sauces and like products, carbonated drinks, non-carbonated drinks including punches and lemonades, concentrated liquids or solids for drinks, beer and malt beverages, snacks including potato, cereal, flour or starch-based (from roots and tubers, pulses and legumes). Composite foods including casseroles, meat pies and mincemeat.'* [115] Further research is needed into manufacture and extraction methods. On alert in the United States and in the European Union. Approved in New Zealand and Australia. **Caution** or **Avoid**

| 363 **Avoid** | Succinic acid |
|---|---|

**Colour: White powder, however the name derives from the Latin meaning amber**
Naturally occurs in some plants and animals. Occurs naturally in fossils, fungi and lichen. Used in gluten-free food as a sweetener. Also used as a growth inhibitor to many strains of bacteria and mould. Used in powdered drinks, puddings, sweets, lollies and confectionary, used in soups, breads and bakery products. Can contribute to food allergies and adverse reactions. *'Negative impact on the brain and nervous system, endocrine disruption and cancer.'* [116] May contribute to skin and eye irritation. Banned in many countries. Approved in the United States and the European Union. Check for approval in New Zealand. Not approved in Australia. **Avoid**

---

[115] http://www.fao.org
[116] http://thearticlebay.com

| 365 | Sodium fumarate |
|---|---|
| **Caution** or **Avoid** | |

**Colour: Odourless, white crystalline powder**
Derived from the plant Fumaria esp F officianalis. Is used as an acidity regulator in processed food, confectionary, bakery products, baking powder. Adds strength to bread dough and greater volume to egg whites or whipped cream. Also used as a lubricant in the manufacturing of tablets and capsules. Fumeric acid and its sodium salts cause body flushes and can damage kidney and kidney function, cause liver damage and damage to the digestive system. On alert in the United States and the European Union. Approved in New Zealand and Australia. **Caution** or **Avoid**

| 366 | Potasium fumerate |
|---|---|
| **Caution** or **Avoid** | |

**Colour: White crystals**
Regulates acidity in jams and preserves. Very little research available. Approved in the United States. On alert in the European Union. Approved in New Zealand and Australia. **Caution** or **Avoid**

| 367 | Calcium fumerate |
|---|---|
| **Caution** or **Avoid** | |

**Colour: Calcium salt**
Is usually a corn derivative used as an acid regulator to enrich foods and boost calcium absorption. Used as a food

additive in commercial products. Added to dietary supplements, beverages, cattle feed and pharmaceutical products. On alert in the United States. Not permitted in the European Union. Approved in New Zealand and Australia. **Caution** or **Avoid**

| 368 **Caution** or **Avoid** | Ammonium fumerate |
|---|---|

**Colour: Chemical compound**
Is a food acid regulator, additive and preservative used in wheat tortillas and like products. May be a substitute for tartaric acid. On alert in the United States. Not permitted in the European Union. Approved in New Zealand and Australia. **Caution** or **Avoid**

| 380 **Avoid** | Tri-ammonium citrate |
|---|---|

**Colour: Reddish-brown powder**
Is an acidity regulator, buffer and emulsifier. Is synthesised by fermentation from sugar beet which is then treated with sulphuric acid which then becomes citric acid and calcium sulphate. Can be extracted by hexane. Is used as a dietary iron supplement in breakfast and dietary formulas. Used in cheese spreads and associated products, chocolates and confectionary. May interfere with liver and pancreas function. *'Is linked to nerve cell destruction, neurological disorders, contains PFGA.'*[117] Linked to additive 620. Can be found in paint emulsions.

---

[117] http://thearticlebay.com (Processed Free Glutamic Acid is a highly dangerous additive)

On alert in the United States. Approved in the European Union, New Zealand and Australia. **Avoid**

| 381 **Caution** | Ferric ammonium citrate |
|---|---|

**Colour: Green-reddish brown powder**
Used as a food additive, anti-caking agent and regulator. Derived from minerals and is a complex mixture of iron, ammonia and citric acid. Is a synthetic of citric acid. Used in dietary and iron supplements, as a supplement in breakfast cereals, Scotch eggs, Irn-Bru and water purification. Approved in the United States. On alert in the European Union. Approved in New Zealand and Australia. **Caution**

| 385 **Avoid** | Calcium disodium ethylenediaminetetraacetate or calcium disodium EDTA |
|---|---|

**Colour: Colourless water-soluble solid**
Used as a food preservative and antioxidant. Is a synthetic and has a synthetic flavour. Used in some imported products into Australia including: canned soft drinks, food dressings, egg products, salads, mayonnaise, dips, sauces, pickles, lima beans, pecan pie fillings, sandwich spreads, imported margarines and tinned white potatoes. Adverse effects of ingesting this additive include: muscle weakness, nausea, vomiting, fainting, dizziness, hypertension, palpitations, gastrointestinal and abdominal pain, muscle cramps, headaches, thrombophlebitis,[118] hypersensitivity, numbness and fever. Linked to: *asthma,*

---

[118] Inflammation of veins.

*kidney damage and kidney disease, liver damage; can increase the absorption of certain toxic heavy metals, cancer, dermatitis and skin rash.'*[119] Can also cause diarrhoea and excessive thirst. Can cause a reduction in natural vitamin intake and mineral imbalance. Banned in some countries. Approved in the United States, European Union, New Zealand and Australia. **Avoid**

---

[119] http://thearticlebay.com

**Your Notes**

......................................................................................

......................................................................................

......................................................................................

......................................................................................

......................................................................................

......................................................................................

......................................................................................

......................................................................................

......................................................................................

......................................................................................

......................................................................................

......................................................................................

......................................................................................

......................................................................................

......................................................................................

......................................................................................

......................................................................................

......................................................................................

......................................................................................

......................................................................................

More research needs to be undertaken to give to the consumer significant information that will allow them to be comfortable when they are making food choices. Colour or traffic lighting the additive numbers would be a good idea but it's doubtful whether food manufacturers would comply with this. That leaves the individual to make their own informed choices.

As you get to know the additive numbers and how some relate to and change behaviour, is it any wonder that children and young adults trying to learn their school subjects have problems when there is so much interference to their brain, mind and body by the food they eat?

## Devils: Vegetable gums, thickeners, stabilisers, emulsifiers and glazing agents (400 range)

| Devil Numbers | Additive |
|:---:|:---:|
| **400** <br> **Caution** or **Avoid** | **Alginic acid** |

**Colour: White to yellow granular powder**

Alginic acid is a natural product of brown seaweed also known as large brown kelp. Used as a thickening agent in jams, jellies, spreads, custard mix, cordial, flavoured milk, ice blocks and ice lollies, pastry, ice cream, cheese, sweets, lollies, thickened cream, confectionary, canned icing, beer thickener, cream and yogurt. In small quantities, no known side effects. People who have allergies to shellfish may have a reaction. In large quantities can restrain the absorption of some nutrients. May be linked to: *'birth defects, severe allergic reaction and neurological disorders.'*[120] Some research has shown it may have the ability to bind with heavy metals in the human system and remove from the body. Approved in the United States, European Union, New Zealand and Australia. **Caution** or **Avoid**

| | |
|:---:|:---:|
| **401** <br> **Caution** or **Avoid** | **Sodium alginate** |

**Colour: White to yellow granular or powder**

Is used as a bulking agent, thickener, stabiliser, foaming , gelling, glazing, emulsifier, humectant and sequestrant in food production. Sodium salt is used in commercially

---

[120] http://thearticlebay.com

247

manufactured bakery and dairy products, food dressings, sauces, in the production of processed meats. In small quantities, no known side effects. As 400, can be linked to: *'birth defects, severe allergic reaction and neurological disorders.'* Some research has shown it may have the ability to bind with heavy metals in the human system and remove them from the body. Approved in the United States, European Union, New Zealand and Australia. **Caution** or **Avoid**

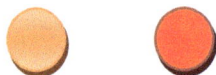

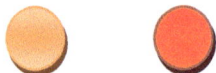

| 402 **Caution** or **Avoid** | Potassium alginate |
|---|---|

**Colour: White powder**
Is used as bulking agent, emulsifier, thickener, stabiliser, glazing, gelling and foaming agent. Derived from seaweed and used in custard mixes, cordials, flavoured milk, ice blocks, thickened cream, yogurt, jam and jelly production. Also used in salad dressings, marmalades, fruit spreads including low-calorie products and antacid preparations. Also used in cottage cheese, processed cheese, cream cheese and icing. As 400, may be linked to: *'birth defects, severe allergic reaction and neurological disorders.'* Some research has shown it may have the ability to bind with heavy metals in the human system and remove from the body. Approved in the United States, European Union, New Zealand and Australia. **Caution** or **Avoid**

| 403 **Caution** or **Avoid** | Ammonium alginate |
|---|---|

**Colour: White to yellow granules powder**
Is natural inorganic emulsifier derived from seaweed and used to thicken food substances. Is used as bulking agent,

emulsifier, thickener, stabiliser, glazing, gelling and foaming agent. Used in custard mixes, cordial drinks, flavoured milk, thickened cream, ice blocks, jams, jellies, marmalades, yogurt, fruit spreads and in low-calorie food production. Also used in antacid medications. In large quantities can inhibit the absorption of other food nutrients. *'Ammonium alginate is recognised as a non-toxic ingredient, but may cause allergic reaction in people who are allergic to shellfish. May affect the respiratory system, gastrointestinal tract and mucus glands.'*[121] As 400, may be linked to: *'birth defects, severe allergic reaction and neurological disorders.'* Approved in the United States, European Union, New Zealand and Australia. **Caution** or **Avoid**

| 404 **Caution** or **Avoid** | Calcium alginate |
|---|---|

**Colour: Cream coloured substance or powder**

Is an emulsifier, thickener, food stabiliser and gelling agent. Is extracted from seaweed and used in manufactured food production. Is used in the production of: ice cream, flavoured milks, jams, jellies, marmalades, ice blocks, artificial sweeteners, slimming aids, cheese production, yogurt and custard powders. Also used in frozen bakery products, thickened cream and indigestion tablets. Large quantities can inhibit the absorption of good food nutrients. Please note: Dietary foods for infants and children for special medical purposes. *'Infants and young children consuming these food categories (400 – 404) may show a higher susceptibility to gastrointestinal salts than their healthy counterparts due to their underlying medical condition.'*[122] As 400, can be linked to: *'birth defects, severe allergic reaction and neurological disorders.'*

---

[121] https://www.naturalpedia.com
[122] https://efsa.onlinelibrary.wiley.com

Approved in the United States, European Union, New Zealand and Australia. Caution or Avoid

| 405 Avoid | Propylene glycol alginate |
|---|---|

**Colour: White to off-white powder**
Can be extracted from the cell walls of brown seaweed or may be extracted by petroleum – check for product source and extraction methods. Is used as a sweetener base, bulking agent, emulsifier, foaming agent, gelling agent, stabiliser and thickener. Used in jellies, marmalades, fruit spreads, yogurt, ice cream. Acts as a stabiliser in milk products including cheeses, cheese spreads, desserts, nut coatings, dairy products, chewing gum and dietary supplements. Also acts as a bubble stabiliser in beer. Added to fruit drinks and as a modifier in flour, noodles and instant foods including ketchup, meat sauces, soy sauce, syrup and icing. Used as a stabiliser in ice cream. Other uses: glazing and sizing of paper, special printer inks, paints, cosmetics, insecticides, germicides, paint remover, anti-freeze; in the production of plastics and in pharmaceutical preparations. Is linked to '*birth defects, severe allergic reactions, neurological disorders.*'[123] Suggested, avoid during pregnancy. Banned in France. Please also see additive 1520. Approved in the United States, European Union, New Zealand and Australia. Avoid

---

[123] http://thearticlebay.com

| 406<br>**Avoid** | **Agar or**<br>**agar agar** |
|---|---|

**Colour: White and semi-translucent powder**

Is a nonorganic, non-synthetic vegetable gum derived from red seaweed. Is a soluble fibre and additive used in pie fillings, meringues, glazing, cream, milk, yogurt, meringue shells, sherbets, ice cream, canned and cured manufactured meats, noodles, cheeses, sauces, baked products, cakes, icings, jelly, candies, sweets, confectionary, fondants and many Asian desserts. Can cause flatulence and distension in the abdomen. '*Is linked to cancer.*[124] Agar, agar approved in the United States, European Union, New Zealand and Australia. **Avoid**

| 407<br>**Avoid** | **Carrageenan** |
|---|---|

**Colour: Extract of red seaweed**

Is a fibre extracted from red seaweed. Used as a vegetable gum, stabiliser, gelling agent and thickener. Is used in preserved meats, including ham, frozen desserts, chocolate, beer, sauces, milk, soy milk, pet food, coffee, beverages, confectionary, sweets, ice creams, yogurts, cheese, cottage cheese, whipping creams, fruit jellies, soft drinks, salad dressings, infant formula, dried pasta products, fish products, vegetarian products, hot dogs and medicines. Is used in air fresheners, gel toothpaste, shampoos and laxatives. Is linked to: '*intestinal disease, intestinal inflammation, severe allergic reactions, negative impact on diseases of the immune system, stomach ulcers, liver damage, delayed growth, birth defects, is a*

---

*neurotoxin, gastro-intestinal cancer, crohn's disease.* [125]
May also be linked to food allergies, food intolerances and
ulcerative colitis. Dr Joanne K. Tobacman, Associate
Professor, published paper from 45 publicly funded
studies, her findings suggest *'the potential role of
carrageenan in the development of gastrointestinal
malignancy and inflammatory bowel disease requires
careful reconsideration of the advisability of its continued
use as a food additive'.* [126] Approved in the United States,
European Union, New Zealand and Australia. **Avoid**

| 409<br>Safe or Caution | Arabinogalactan or larch gum |
|---|---|

**Colour: Sold in powder form**
Is a polysaccharide,[127] larch gum extracted by water from
larch wood. Is used as a thickener in manufactured foods.
Also used in chewable tablets, chewing gum and bakery
products. Is used in confectionary, chocolates, frozen milk-
based drinks and mustard. Also used in the pharmaceutical
industry in medicines. It appears to increase the immune
system. *'The safety of Arabinogalactan is supported by its
daily consumption in common fruits and vegetables, its
fermentation by bacteria in the human colon and its ability
to rapidly signal faecal bacteria enzymes to begin the
fermentation process.* [128] Is also used in animal feed, pulp
production, oil production and other combinations within
industrial production. Approved in the United States. On
alert in the European Union. Approved in New Zealand and
Australia. **Safe** or **Caution**

---

[125] http://thearticlebay.com
[126] https://www.naturalhealthmag.com.au
[127] A carbohydrate whose molecules have a number of sugar
molecules bond as one.
[128] https://infogalactic.com

| 410<br>**Caution** | **Locust bean gum or<br>carob bean gum** |
|---|---|

**Colour: White to yellowish powder**
Is a vegetable gum extract from the seeds of the carob tree, Ceratonia siliqua. Is used in low-fat foods, biscuits or cookies and ice cream, Is also used to thicken frozen desserts, cultured dairy products, baked goods, dried fruit and liqueurs, vodka, sweets and confectionary, soft drinks, toothpaste and marshmallows. Used in cream cheese, frozen desserts and dairy products. Also used as a thickener, artificial sweetener base, stabiliser in lollies, sweets, some confectionary, cordials, essences, flour products, fruit juice. Used in caffeine-free chocolate. May lower cholesterol. Can cause allergic reactions including skin reaction, asthma and hay fever. Also abdominal pain, diarrhoea and coughs in infants. Approved in the United States, European Union, New Zealand and Australia. **Caution**

| 412<br>**Caution** or **Avoid** | **Guar gum** |
|---|---|

**Colour: White to light yellow free-flowing powder**
Used as a thickener and stabiliser. A gum derived from the seeds of the Cyamoposis tetragonolobus bean. Used in ice cream, dairy products, processed meat, dressings, sauces, cereal, fruit drinks, frozen fruit, cheese spread, jellies and preserves, including jam, yogurt-based products, kefir (fermented milk drink) and sauces. Widely used in the bakery industry. Is also used as a stabiliser in chocolate and fruit drinks. Linked to: '*delayed growth, intestinal inflammation, intestinal disorders, cancer, endocrine disruption, severe allergic reactions, enlarged thyroid gland, bloating, severe allergic reactions, enlargement of*

*the thyroid gland.*[129] Found in many organic foods. Can add to weight gain. Allowed by the Swedish KRAV.[130] Approved in the United States, European Union, New Zealand and Australia. **Caution** or **Avoid**

| 413 **Avoid** | Tragacanth gum |
|---|---|

**Colour: White to pale yellow fragments**
Is a natural gum produced from the tree Astragalus, gummifer. Is used as an emulsifier, stabiliser, and thickener. Used in salad dressing, cream cheese, ice creams, icing and cottage cheese. Also used in drugs, nasal solutions, tablets and elixirs. May be linked to asthma, skin rashes, gastrointestinal disorders and dermatitis. Also linked to: *'liver damage, miscarriages, severe allergic reactions, rash and laxative.'*[131] Approved in the United States, European Union, New Zealand and Australia. **Avoid**

| 414 **Avoid** | Gum Arabic or Acacia gum |
|---|---|

**Colour: gold to brown hardened sap**
A natural gum made of hardened sap from two species of Acacia. Used as a thickener, stabiliser, glazing agent and emulsifier. Also used in the manufacture of marshmallows, soft drinks, chewing gum, jelly, fondants, hard gummy lollies, sweets, confectionary, beer, soft drinks, fruit drinks/squash, wine and syrups. Also found in health foods

---

[129] http://thearticlebay.com
[130] Certification Body of Organic Products.
[131] http://thearticlebay.com

including organic chocolate, covered nuts and lollies, sweets or candies. Can cause: Asthma, skin rashes and flatulence. Also linked to: *'birth defects, severe asthma attacks, cancer, severe reactions.'*[132] May assist with soothing irritation to mucous membranes. Approved in the United States, European Union, New Zealand and Australia. **Avoid**

| 415  Caution | Xanthan Gum |
|---|---|

**Colour: Fine white powder**
Is a common food additive used as an emulsifier, foaming agent, stabiliser and thickening agent. Can be genetically modified from corn sugar. Is produced by the process of fermenting glucose or sucrose with the micro-organism: Xanthomonas campestris. Foods containing Xanthan gum include: breads and baked goods, dairy and thickened dairy foods, creamed condiments, canned meats, paté and salad dressing. Is also used to emulsify oil. Also used in some animal feeds. May contribute to skin irritation, hay fever, asthma, bloating, cramps and flatulence. Approved in the United States, European Union, New Zealand and Australia. **Caution**

---

[132] http://thearticlebay.com

| 416 Caution or Avoid | Karaya gum |
|---|---|

**Colour: Pale grey to pinkish grey**
Is a processed vegetable gum obtained from the tree Sterculia uren. Often used with carob. Has the ability to multiply the volume of ingredients up to 100 percent. Is used in potato and cereal-based snacks, bakery products, cheese, custards, ice cream, spreads, desserts, nut coatings and fillings, emulsified sauces, dietary food supplements, egg-based liqueurs, dairy products, chewing gum, sweets, lollies, confectionary and in laxatives. Also used as a denture adhesive. Is a possible allergen known to cause allergic reactions, urticaria, asthma and dermatitis. May cause adverse reactions including *intestinal cancer.*[133] Approved in the United States, European Union, New Zealand and Australia. Caution or Avoid

| 417 Caution or Avoid | Tara gum |
|---|---|

**Colour: Beige to yellow to white, almost odourless powder**
Is used as a thickener, stabiliser, foaming, emulsifying and gelling agent. Obtained from the seeds of the Caesalpinia spinosa tree. Used in bakery products, baked goods, dehydrated foods, salad dressing, canned meats, jellies, jams, mouse, yogurt, cheese, fruit juices, cakes, mustards, pickles, candies, lollies, sweets, mayonnaise, cocoa-based drinks, sauces, ice cream and soft drinks. High concentrations bring about bloating and flatulence,

---

[133] http://thearticlebay.com

intestinal distress, gas, loose stools and diarrhoea. May contribute to severe allergic reactions including skin rashes, hives, chest tightness, shortness in breath, coughing, wheezing, watery eyes, runny nose, stomach cramps, vomiting and nausea. May contribute to '*intestinal cancer*' (the Article Bay). On alert in the United States. Approved in the European Union. New Zealand and Australia. **Caution** or **Avoid**

| 418 **Caution** or **Avoid** | Gellan gum |
|---|---|

**Colour: White or off-white powder**
Identified in 1978 from the tissue of lily plants in the United States. Is used as an emulsifier, suspension agent, stabilizer gelling agent and thickener. Used in jams, candy, sweets and confectionary, desserts, ice cream, sorbets and dairy products. Used in soy milk to keep the soy protein suspended. Also used in flour. Is used in beverages, animal feed and in other industries. Extreme intake may cause excessive gas, (flatulence) abdominal bloating and discomfort, loose or enlarged stools, diarrhoea and nausea. May also contribute to '*intestinal cancer, intestinal inflammation and severe allergic reactions.*[134] Concerns have been raised about this product's use with new born babies and its use in infant and young children's food. On alert in the United States. Approved in Japan, European Union, Canada, China, Korea, New Zealand and Australia. **Caution** or **Avoid**

---

[134] http://thearticlebay.com

**Your Notes**

.......................................................................

.......................................................................

.......................................................................

.......................................................................

.......................................................................

.......................................................................

.......................................................................

.......................................................................

.......................................................................

.......................................................................

.......................................................................

.......................................................................

.......................................................................

.......................................................................

.......................................................................

.......................................................................

.......................................................................

.......................................................................

.......................................................................

**Devils: Humectants also used as sweeteners (400 range)**

| Devil Numbers | Additive |
|:---:|:---:|
| 420<br>Caution or Avoid | Sorbitol or sorbitol syrup and Sorbitol (i) and(ii) |

**Colour: White crystalline odourless powder**

Is an artificial sweetener and humectant.[135] Is derived from berries of the Rowan or Mountain Ash tree or can be synthesised. It is a sugar alcohol. Is used as a bulking agent in a variety of foods. Used in low-calorie foods, bacon, breads, cakes, cheese, chewing gum, cookies or biscuits, drinks, gluten-free ingredients, ice cream, puddings, sauces, sausages, whiskey, wine, pastries, confectionary, dried fruits, pastries, mint sweets and lollies, juices and pharmaceutical syrups. Is widely used in diabetic food. Can cause gastric disturbance and stomach distension. Sorbitols may be linked to: *'eye injuries, intestinal disorders, severe allergic reactions, diarrhoea, kidney stones, kidney tumours and cramps.*[136] Not permitted in foods for infants and young children. Approved in the United States, European Union, New Zealand and Australia. Caution or Avoid

---

[135] Humectants – keep food moist and allows for a longer shelf life in cakes, bread, rolls and other baked foods bought at the bakery.
[136] http://thearticlebay.com

| 421 **Avoid** | Mannitol |
|---|---|

**Colour: White crystalline organic compound**

Is a natural carbohydrate present in conifer, mushrooms, Manna ash tree and seaweed. Commercially it's a sugar which is produced by hydrogenation[137] of invert sugar. Is used as an anti-caking, low calorie, bulking agent. Is used in sugar-free foods; it retains moisture in baked goods, mustards, puddings, bakery products, confectionary, sauces and frozen fish. Can cause nausea, intestinal disorder, severe allergic reactions, bloating, diarrhoea, vomiting, kidney dysfunction and damage, kidney disease and cancer. Not for diabetics. Not permitted in infant or young children's food. Not recommended for those people with kidney or liver impairment. Other names: Hexanehexol, mannite, manna sugar. Approved in the United States, European Union, New Zealand and Australia. **Avoid**

| 422 **Caution** or **Avoid** | Glycerine or glycerol |
|---|---|

**Colour: Colourless, odourless, sweet oily, colourless alcohol**

Is a synthetic product derived from decomposition of natural fats with alkalis and a by-product of soap production and manufacturing. Can be obtained from petroleum or synthesised propylene. Is used as a sweetener and preservative for foods. Is also used as a filler in low-fat foods. Used in e-cigarettes and in the flexible coating on sausages and used in cheese production

---

[137] Treated with hydrogen through the use of either: heated nickel, palladium or platinum rods; a dangerous process for food.

also in crystallised and dried fruit, in vodka, liqueurs, soft drinks, marshmallows, sweets and confectionary, baked goods, toothpaste and other products. Is linked to: *'endocrine disruption, reproductive disorder, kidney disorders and cancer.'*[138] Large quantities can cause high blood sugar, thirst, headaches and nausea. Natural glycerine may protect DNA against tumour development. More research needed on this additive. Approved in the United States, European Union, New Zealand and Australia. **Caution** or **Avoid**

---

[138] http://thearticlebay.com

**Your Notes**

........................................................................

........................................................................

........................................................................

........................................................................

........................................................................

........................................................................

........................................................................

........................................................................

........................................................................

........................................................................

........................................................................

........................................................................

........................................................................

........................................................................

........................................................................

........................................................................

........................................................................

........................................................................

# Devils: Emulsifiers (400 range)

| Devil Numbers | Additive |
|:---:|:---:|
| **431** <br> **Avoid** | **Polyoxyethylene (40) stearate** |

**Colour: Cream coloured flakes or faint colour in waxy solid**

A synthetic compound produced by a reaction of ethylene oxide[139] with stearic acid.[140] Used as an emulsifier and stabiliser in manufactured bread and pudding production. Ethylene oxide is made from gas and petroleum and is used in detergent production. Is linked to liver damage, skin disorder, urinary tract problems, eczema, cancer, kidney and liver damage. Approved in the United States, European Union, New Zealand and Australia. **Avoid**

| Devil Numbers | Additive |
|:---:|:---:|
| **433** <br> **Avoid** | **Polysorbate 80 or Polyoxyethylene (20) sorbitan monooleate or PEG 80** |

**Colour: Lemon to amber**

Is a synthetic additive derived from esterification[141] of polyethoxylated sorbitan and oleic acid. Used in synthetic flavourings as a de-foaming agent and to condition dough used in commercial food production including cupcake mixes, instant pasta, pie topping and pie tops, sauces, muesli bars, ice cream and instant soups. Also used in chewing gum, ice cream and soft drinks. Can irritate mucous membranes, upper respiratory tract, also linked to

---

[139] A flammable toxic gas.

[140] A solid saturated fatty acid from either vegetable or animal fats.

[141] Esters are derived from carboxylic acid and alcohol.

intestinal disorders, eczema, kidney and liver damage and cancer. '*Is linked to miscarriage and infertility.*'[142] Approved in the United States, European Union, New Zealand, banned in Australia. **Avoid**

| 435 **Avoid** | Polysorbate 60 or Polyoxyethylene (20) Sorbitan monostearate or Peg 60 |
|---|---|

**Colour: Lemon to orange oily liquid**

Is a synthetic compound and known by two other names: polysorbate 60 and peg 60. Is a derivative of sorbitol, ethylene oxide as a petroleum and stearic acid. Is used as a emulsifier, gelling agent, stabilisers and thickener. Is used in synthetic flavourings, surfactants.[143] Used as a foaming agent and conditioner in commercially made dough products. Prevents baked goods from going stale, helps coffee whiteners dissolve in coffee and stops the oil from separating in whipped cream. Found in bakery products, frozen desserts, imitation dairy products, soups, sauces, bread, cakes, crisps, spreads, jam, chocolate, margarine, quick setting desserts and milk shakes. Is linked to: '*intestinal disorders, eczema, cancer, kidney and liver damage.*'[144] Can cause abdominal distension, flatulence and diarrhoea. Harmful through ingestion and inhalation. May cause irritation in mucous membranes and the respiratory tract. Can also cause irritation to skin and eyes. Approved in the United States, European Union, New Zealand and Australia. **Avoid**

---

[142] http://www.wotzinurfood.com
[143] Lowers the surface tension between liquids or between liquids and solids.
[144] http://thearticlebay.com

| 436<br>**Avoid** | **Polysorbate 65 or Polyoxyethylene (20) sorbitan tristearate** |
|---|---|

**Colour: Tan coloured waxy solid**
Is a synthetic compound produced from ethylene oxide,[145] a petroleum derivative. Is used as a food emulsifier and food stabiliser. Also used in aerosol sprays, long-life milk, low-calorie cream, pasteurised products and laxatives. Is used in cake fillings, cake mixes, cakes, frozen desserts, ice cream, chewing gum, imitation dairy products, frozen desserts, emulsified soups and sauces, bakery products, soft drinks, coffee substitutes and a wide range of detergents. Can cause flatulence, diarrhoea, abdominal distension. Also linked to: *'intestinal disorders, eczema, cancer, kidney damage and liver damage.'* See thearticlebay.com. Can irritate mucous membranes and the upper respiratory tract. Is a suspected carcinogen. May also cause irritation to eyes and skin. Approved in the United States, European Union, New Zealand and Australia. **Avoid**

| 440<br>**Caution** or **Avoid** | **Pectin** |
|---|---|

**Colour: White to light brown powder**
Pectin is a naturally occurring gelling agent or polysaccharide found in many ripe fruits including the skins of apples, blackberries, oranges, plums and citrus fruits. Commercially manufactured pectin is a gelling, thickening and stabilising agent used in confectionary, sweets, jams, preserves and acid milk drinks. It may cause intestinal problems and flatulence when ingested in high

---

[145] Ethylene oxide is industrially produced by oxidation.

concentrations. Commercial pectin may contain unbound glutamic acid or (PFGA). *'One cannot compare naturally bound glutamic acid with a man-made chemically processed, isolated, unbound amino acid which is full of dangerous contaminants.'*[146] For more information on this food additive number, please see[147] and the references to 620-625. Check the label before purchase. Approved in the United States, European Union, New Zealand and Australia. **Caution** or **Avoid**

| 442 **Avoid** | Ammonium salts of phosphatidic acid Soy lecithin |
|---|---|

**Colour: White crystal**
Obtained mainly from the fatty acids of rape seed oil[148] and ammonia fatty acids. Of all of the oils produced, rape seed is the most toxic as the majority is extracted using hexane a petroleum-based product. Ammonium phosphatide/soy lecithin is used in the production of cocoa and a wide range of highly branded, with worldwide distribution, chocolate products, chocolate spreads and other chocolate and related products including confectionary, cakes, biscuits, sweets, lollies and food with chocolate added. Can leach calcium from the human body. Some outcomes lead to low blood pressure, fainting, dizziness, nausea, abdominal pain, excessive weight gain, bloating, coughing, excessive perspiration, blurred vision, shock, anaphylactic shock and in severe cases, death. Is linked to: *'nerve cell destruction and kidney disorders.'*[149] This product is used in food, clothing and cosmetics. More research is required on this product.

---

[146] http://thearticlebay.com
[147] www.truthinlabeling.org
[148] Rapeseed oil contains high levels ferulic acid – in large amounts can be toxic to the human body.
[149] http://thearticlebay.com

On alert in the United States. Approved in the European Union. Banned in New Zealand and Australia. **Avoid**

| 444 **Avoid** | Sucrose acetate isobutyrate |
|---|---|

**Colour: Tasteless light yellow liquid**
Is a synthetic food product derived from cane sugar. Is used as an emulsifier and food stabiliser. Used in pasteurised products, ice creams, cheeses, dairy products, batters, spreads, breakfast cereals and bakery goods including: breads and dough products. Also used in flavouring oils and non-alcoholic cloudy and flavoured drinks. May cause respiratory, digestive tract irritation and intestinal disorders. In animal studies and in high doses, it shows brain and nervous system negative behavioural effects. It may be a neurotoxin.[150] It is suspect and may be an environmental toxin. With persistent use, within the human body, it may lead to toxin accumulation. Approved in the United States, European Union, New Zealand and Australia. **Avoid**

---

[150] Toxins destructive to nerve tissue.

| 445<br>**Avoid** | **Glycerol esters of rosin**<br>**Glycerol esters of gum rosin (i)**<br>**Glycerol esters of tall oil rosin (ii)**<br>**Glycerol esters of wood rosins (iii)** |
|---|---|

**Colour: Pine resin**

Extracted by the solvent methanol from the stumps of long-leaf pine (Pinus Palustris). Used in pasteurised products including: cheeses, ice cream, batters, dairy products, breakfast cereals, spreads, orange fizzy, canned drinks and bakery goods. '*High intakes may upset calcium and phosphate equilibrium, cause vomiting, headaches, dehydration, thirst, diarrhoea, dizziness and mental confusion.*'[151] Is linked to: '*skin blisters, rashes, flaky skin, itchy skin*'.[152] May increase liver size and raise sugar levels. Also known to increase eye irritation in sensitive people. Used in low-cost adhesives. Listed under Additive Alert.[153] More research needed. Approved in the United States, 455, (i), (ii), (iii). Approved in the European Union 455. On alert in the European Union (i), (ii), (iii). Approved in New Zealand and Australia 455. On alert in Australia (i), (ii), (iii). **Avoid**

---

[151] https://noshly.com

[152] http://thearticlebay.com

[153] http://doi.org/10.2903/j.efsa.2018.537

**Your Notes**

..................................................................................

..................................................................................

..................................................................................

..................................................................................

..................................................................................

..................................................................................

..................................................................................

..................................................................................

..................................................................................

..................................................................................

..................................................................................

..................................................................................

..................................................................................

..................................................................................

..................................................................................

..................................................................................

..................................................................................

..................................................................................

..................................................................................

# Devils: More mineral salts (400 range)

| Devil Numbers | Additive |
|---|---|
| 450<br>Caution or Avoid | Diphosphates<br>(i) Disodium diphosphate<br>(ii) Trisodium diphosphate<br>(iii) Tetrasodium diphosphate<br>(iv) Dipotassium diphosphate<br>(v) Tetrapotassium diphosphate<br>(vi) Dicalcium diphosphate<br>(vii) Calcium dihydrogen diphosphate<br>(viii)Dimagnesium diphosphate<br>(ix) Magnesium dihydrogen diphosphate |

**Colour: Colourless or white crystals**

Is a synthetic substance produced from individual carbonates and phosphoric acid. Is used as a food stabiliser, acidity regulator, emulsifier, raising agent and sequestrant.[154] In Europe, may be derived from animal bones. Used as a bread and product enhancer. Used in the metal industry to bind metal and stop discolouration. *'High intake may upset the calcium/phosphate equilibrium and excessive use may lead to osteoporosis.'*[155] Diphosphates are *'linked to kidney damage and kidney disease, disorder of the digestive system, intestinal disorders, may impair the body's ability to absorb minerals.'*[156] Always check the

---

[154] A substance which control the metal ions in copper, iron and nickel. These prevent the oxidation of fats in foods.
[155] http://www.wotzinurfood.com
[156] http://thearticlebay.com

450 number. Approved in the United States. On alert in the United States (iv). Approved in the European Union. On alert in the European Union (iv) and (viii). Approved in New Zealand and Australia. On alert in New Zealand and Australia (iv) and (viii) **Caution** or **Avoid**

| 451 **Avoid** | Potassium triphosphates **(i) Pentasodium triphosphate** **(ii) Pentapotassium triphosphate** |
|---|---|

**Colour: White granules or powder**
Are salts of sodium and potassium with phosphates. In Europe obtained from animal bones. In the United States, obtained from minerals. Used in processed rainwater and in cured meats such as ham. High intakes may upset the equilibrium of the human body and can lead to osteoporosis. Is also known to cause nausea, diarrhoea, lowers blood pressure, cyanosis[157] and muscle spasms. May cause intestinal disorders, harm the body's ability to absorb minerals, cause disorders to the digestive system leading to kidney damage and disease. All on alert in the United States, in the European Union, New Zealand and Australia. **Avoid**

---

[157] A bluish discolouration of the skin.

| 452<br>Avoid | Potassium polymetaphosphate<br>(i) Sodium phosphate<br>(ii) Potassium phosphate<br>(iii) Sodium calcium phosphate<br>(iv) Calcium phosphate<br>(v) Ammonium phosphate<br>(vi) Sodium potassium tripolyphosphate |
|---|---|

**Colour: Colourless crystals or granular powder**

Potassium polymetaphosphate are the salts of sodium, potassium and calcium combined with phosphate. Is a gluten-free additive. Is used as a stabilizer, thickener and to regulate moisture. Often used in soft and alcoholic drinks, fresh and canned meats including sausages, ham and dried vegetables. Also used in chewing gum, chocolate, cereals, candy sweets, dairy and commercially baked products. Also found in gammon, German, soft cheese, cut pork, processed cheese, commercially manufactured meat pies and many soft fruit drinks. Can change the metabolic activity in humans. In animal studies has proven to increase the calcification of the pelvic area in rats. May intensify the absorption of heavy metals making them easier to penetrate the intestinal wall. Is linked to: 'kidney damage and disease, disorders of the digestive system, intestinal disorders; may impair the body's ability to absorb minerals.'[158] All on alert in United States and in the European Union. Only one approved in New Zealand and Australia (i) sodium phosphate. **Avoid**

---

[158] http://thearticlebay.com

**Your Notes**

## Devils: Thickeners (400 range)

| Devil Numbers | Additive |
|---|---|
| **460**<br>Caution or Avoid | **Cellulose microcrystalline and Cellulose powdered** |

**Colour: Fine white powder**
Is natural and inorganic. Refined from wood pulp and genetically modified cotton stems. May be derived from genetically modified crops. Is used as an anti-caking agent, texture creator, fat substitute and bulking agent in the food industry. Is commonly used in vitamins and supplements. Also used in fermented milk products, flavoured milk, unflavoured cream and related products. Also used in fermented cream and related products including: unripened cheese, margarine, ripened cheese, whey, processed cheese, jams, chocolate, quick setting desserts, beverage whiteners, tinned aerosol vegetable oil spray, sauces, breads, soups, biscuits and cakes. Is added to frozen different desserts, ice blocks, lollies and milk shakes. Banned in the United Kingdom in baby food. May lead to gas and bloating. May contain dioxin.[159] Can increase the absorption of certain toxic heavy metals in the human body. May cause birth defects. Should not be given to infants. Can cause intestinal problems including: bloating, constipation and diarrhoea. Approved in the United States, European Union, New Zealand and Australia. **Caution** or **Avoid**

---

[159] Substances are by products of combustion and various industrial processes such as chlorine bleaching of paper pulp and smelting. World Health Organisation. (WHO)

| 461 **Avoid** | Methyl cellulose |
|---|---|

**Colour: Hydrophilic white powder in pure form**

Is synthetic additive which is commercially prepared from wood and cotton products. Can be chemically methylated, a by-product of petroleum. Is chemically modified and may contain dioxin. Used as a thickening agent, anti-clamping agent, emulsifier and gelling agent. Also used as a filler in dietary fibre. Used in imitation cream, imitation ice cream. Also used in bakery products, dairy-based drinks, yogurts, edible ices and ice cream products, batters, cereals, diabetic and low calorie foods, soft and fizzy drinks, jams, jellies, baked foods, sauces, breads, biscuits, cakes, margarine, crisps, spreads, chocolate, quick setting desserts, sauces, fizzy drinks and many other foods. Can cause flatulence, distension, intestinal disorders and obstruction. Severe allergic reaction. May increase the absorption of some toxic heavy metals in the human body. *'Is linked to cancer. Please note: often in vitamins, minerals and herbs which are sold in ordinary shops and health food stores.'*[160] Approved in the United States, European Union, New Zealand and Australia. **Avoid**

| 463 **Avoid** | Hydroxypropyl cellulose |
|---|---|

**Colour: Light yellow to grey odourless, tasteless, granular or fibrous powder**

Is a synthetic product prepared from wood which is chemically ethylated and a by-product of petroleum that has adverse effects on the human body. May also be a

---

[160] http://thearticlebay.com

derivative of genetically modified cotton. Is used as a thickening agent in many products including dietary products. Is found in dairy and fruit-based desserts, cereals, heat treated meat, chewing gum, dairy drinks, cocoa mixes, weight reduction formulas and electrolyte drinks. May cause intestinal problems, including bloating or gas formation, constipation and diarrhoea. May be linked to digestive problems and cancer. Approved in the United States and the European Union. On alert in Australia. **Avoid**

| 464<br>**Avoid** | Hydroxypropyl methyl cellulose |
|---|---|

**Colour: White powder**
Is commercially prepared from wood and chemically modified with propylene oxide – a plastic and petroleum-based product. In food it's use is in milk for baby formulas, milk powders, icings, coffee, chewing gum, coffee whiteners, bakery products including cakes, pasty products, butter and cake mixes, pasteurised cream, low-calorie cream, pasteurised low-fat cream and pro-biotic multi-vitamins. Has many uses in other industries: tile adhesive, cement renders, gypsum products, paints and coatings, detergents and cleaners, eye drops and contact lenses. Large concentrations can cause, diarrhoea, bloating, constipation, digestive problems, gas formation and endocrine disruption. Approved in the United States, European Union, New Zealand and Australia. **Avoid**

| 465 **Avoid** | Methyl ethyl cellulose |
|---|---|

**Colour: Slightly yellowish odourless powder**
Is a by-product of genetically modified cotton and wood products. To meet the mass-market demand is chemically methylated and ethylated with dimethyl sulphate, (a colourless liquid) and ethyl chloride. These products are a by-product of petroleum. Petroleum has adverse effects on the human system and body. Used as a thickener agent, foaming agent, stabiliser and emulsifier in food production. Used in cheaper chocolate, as a cocoa butter substitute. Also used in cake mixes, toppings, icing, low-fat spreads, salad dressing and chocolate lollies. Is used for imitation cream and ice cream. Is not very soluble and ferments in the large intestine. Is linked to: *'digestive problems, gas formation, bloating, constipation, diarrhoea and cancer.'*[161] Approved in the United States, European Union, New Zealand and Australia. **Avoid**

| 466 **Avoid** | Sodium carboxy methyl-cellulose Cellulose gum (CMC) |
|---|---|

**Colour: White to yellow granules**
Is commercially and chemically prepared from wood and other plant material. Is a synthetic product which is chemically methylated and ethylated which is a by-product of petroleum. May also be a product of genetically modified cotton. Is used as a bulking agent, thickener, stabiliser, foaming, gelling, glazing, emulsifier and humectant in food production. Used in thickeners, emulsifiers, in bakery products, soft drinks, ice cream, long-life milk, low-calorie cream, pasteurised low-fat cream and processed meats.

---

[161] http://thearticlebay.com

Found in tablets and capsules, packaged vitamins and minerals, herb products which are sold in health food shops and other commercial outlets. Also used in tobacco, detergents, toothpaste and paint. Large concentrations can cause intestinal problems, bloating, constipation and diarrhoea. Linked to cancer. The National Cancer Institute of America states: '*It should be forbidden as a food additive 466.*'[162] 466-469 are highly dangerous additives. Approved in the United States, European Union, New Zealand and Australia. **Avoid**

---

[162] http://www.wotzinurfood.com

**Your Notes**

............................................................................

............................................................................

............................................................................

............................................................................

............................................................................

............................................................................

............................................................................

............................................................................

............................................................................

............................................................................

............................................................................

............................................................................

............................................................................

............................................................................

............................................................................

............................................................................

............................................................................

............................................................................

............................................................................

............................................................................

**Devils: Emulsifiers (400 range)**

Please note: fatty acids have a reputation for being part of a healthy diet they can be far from healthy!

'*Many fatty acids and their counterparts are extracted using many levels of petroleum-based chemicals including: ether, hexane and tetrachloroethylene which are considered a known caricinogen. These chemicals are harmful to the body but they are used in bread which is labelled as fatty acids, which are considered healthy, which is potentially misleading to the general public.*'[163]

Despite assumptions or comments made, once ingested, many toxins or poisons cannot leave the human body; they are with you for life. While continually consuming food with these additives they will continue to build up within your body's system and may promote long-term illness.

---

[163] http://www.wotzinurfood.com

# Devils: More emulsifiers (400 range) Emulsifiers

| Devil Numbers | Additive |
|:---:|:---:|
| 470<br>Avoid | Salts of fatty acids salts of aluminium, ammonia, calcium, magnesium, potassium and sodium<br>Also known as:<br>(i) Salts of myristic, palmitic and stearic acids with ammonia, calcium, potassium and sodium<br>(ii) Salts of oleic acid with calcium, potassium and sodium<br>(iii)Magnesium stearate |

**Colour: Hard white and faintly yellowish**
Produced from either plant or animal (pork) origin. Fatty acids from either plant or animal are chemically the same. The acids are a combination of oleic,[164] stearic,[165] myristinic[166] and palmitic acids.[167] Is used as an emulsifier, gelling agent, stabiliser, artificial sweetener and as an anti-caking, release agent. Used in cake mixes, oven-ready chips and in many commercially manufactured food products. Also used in vitamins, minerals and herbs sold in many different commercial outlets. Added to cosmetics, plant dye and soap production. Can irritate the bowel lining, weaken the immune system, damage the intestines, contribute to liver disorders and disrupt the endocrine system. Banned in some countries. Check product labels.

---

[164] Is a non-essential fatty acid – the human body produces what it needs.
[165] Stearic acid is a long-chain fatty acid with up to 18 carbon links within the chain.
[166] Is a long-chain fatty acid mainly found in milk and vegetables.
[167] A by-product of palm oil that may cause cancer.

Approved in the United States. Approved in the European Union, on alert Magenesium stearate (iii). Approved in New Zealand and Australia. On alert Magenesium stearate (iii). **Avoid**

| 471 **Avoid** | Mono- and di-glycerides of fatty acids |
|---|---|

**Colour: White to cream wax solid also in flakes**
Synthetic fats produced from glyceryl and fatty acids primarily from hydrogenated soybean oil. May also come from pork extraction. Fatty acids are extracted by various means including the use of petroleum. Additional acids may include: stearic, oleic, palmitic, and myristinic. Toxicities vary by the extraction methods used. Is used as a thickening agent and emulsifier. Used in cake mixes, black forest gateau, nuts, hot chocolate mixes, fruits, bread mousses, margarine, dessert toppings, cheesecakes, aerosol creams, low fat cream, sponge puddings and oven-ready chips. Used to extend food shelf life. Is used in the lubrication industry Is linked to *'birth defects, cancer and genetic damage.'*[168] On alert in the United States. Approved in the European Union and New Zealand. Banned in Australia. **Avoid**

| 472a **Avoid** | Acetic and fatty acid esters of glycerol |
|---|---|

**Colour: Colour less liquid**
A synthetic solution prepared commercially from glycerine (422) and fatty acids normally obtained from soybean oil which may be genetically modified. May also be from

---
[168] http://thearticlebay.com

animal origin, possibly pork. May have different levels of toxicity depending on the extraction method used. Fatty acids can be extracted by the use of many different levels of petroleum-based chemicals including tetrachloroethylene and hexane which are considered carcinogens. Improves aeration in pastry, and cakes and high fat baking. Is also found in bread, biscuits, cheesecakes, dessert toppings, commercially baked products, dairy foods, edible fats, whipped fats, meat products, margarine, mousse mixes, whipping cream, ice cream, ice cream whitener and salad dressings. Used in wheat-based bread which gives the product the home baked taste and appeal. Is used in brand leading chocolate bars which are sold in the worldwide marketplace. Using this additive allows manufacturers to cut the cost of production. Can protect from moisture loss in sausages. Is capable of forming a thin, flexible film over food products. Is also used to coat meat products, nuts and fruit. Used in Chinese food, preserved pickles, vegetables, beetroot and gherkins, mint sauce, sushi rice, fish sticks, cooking oils, flours and French fries. Can extend shelf life up to 18 months. Can interfere with intestinal workings, diarrhoea, mental confusion, dizziness and thirst. Is linked to: *'injuries to the testicles and reduced sperm production.'*[169] On alert in the United States. Approved in the European Union, New Zealand and Australia. **Avoid**

| 472b **Avoid** | Lactic and fatty acid esters of glycerol |
|---|---|
| **Colour: Cream with fluid powder** Acetic acids mainly from different synthetic fats produced from glycerol and fatty acids. Occurs mainly from plant origins including nuts and fruit skins. May also be derived from animal fat (pork). Is a mixture of acetic, lactic, ||

---

[169] http://thearticlebay.com

tartaric and citric acids. Processing is all down to the method of extraction used. Many fatty acids are extracted using petroleum-based chemicals, some considered carcinogen. Can be genetically modified. These chemicals are harmful to the human body. Labelled as fatty acids, they are used in breads of all types which can be misleading to the general public. Other uses: *'dairy foods, margarine, ice cream, wheat-based bakery goods which have a home-baked taste, and many meat products.'*[170] Also used in oven-ready chips. Used in worldwide brand chocolate. 472b is a mixture of emulsifiers, stabiliser, plasticisers and surface active agents. May cause headaches, nausea, interfere with intestinal functions, vomiting, thirst, dehydration, diarrhoea, dizziness and mental confusion. Is linked to: *'birth defects, cancer and genetic damage.'*[171] On alert in the United States. Approved in the European Union, New Zealand and Australia. Avoid

| 472c  Avoid | Citric and fatty acid esters of glycerol |
|---|---|

**Colour: White to ivory waxy product**
Is a synthetic chemically made (possibly from palm oil), processed fatty acid from unbound amino acids. This additive can be full of dangerous contaminants which form PFGA.[172] Many fatty acids and their equivalents are produced using many levels of petroleum-based chemicals including: ether, tetrachloroethylene, (which is considered to be a known carcinogen) and hexane. This is a highly refined, manufactured poison containing D-glutamic acid (a proven neuro-poison). Amino acid is naturally occurring,

---

[170] http://www.wotzinurfood.com
[171] http://thearticlebay.com
[172] Processed free glutamic acid (PFGA) is highly refined and unbound to amino acids, please see 620.

naturally bound acid found in many naturally grown foods. The range of 472, additives are not natural products and can be produced from other sources including animal. 472c is added to dairy products, batters, sponge cakes, Swiss rolls made from starch, flour and eggs; cake mixes, oven-ready chips, a variety of breads and bakery products including cakes, bread mixes, margarine, ice cream, many wheat-based products, edible fats, (making non-splash in frying oils and products), whipped fats, cooking oils, mayonnaise, salad dressings, low-calorie foods. Is used as a meat binder in sausages and used in many meat products. To cut production costs, is used in world brand chocolate products. Is also used as a protein-binding agent in flour and decreases oil content in dough. Is used as a coating agent in many products, texture modifier, solvent and lubricant. Contributes to many health conditions including: Attention Deficit Disorder (ADD), Attention Deficit Hyperactivity Disorder (ADHD), obesity, convulsions, Chinese Restaurant Disorder (CRS), sweating and dizziness, facial swelling and other health conditions. For more information please see, http://thearticlebay.com. On alert in the United States. Approved in the European Union, New Zealand and Australia. **Avoid**

| 472e<br>**Avoid** | **Diacetyltartaric and fatty acid esters of glycerol** |
|---|---|

**Colour: Cream white fluid powder**
Is linked to the 472 range of addititives. May be an extract of palm oil (palm oil has over 200 different names, please see page 65). Can also be extracted from genetically modified soya beans. Are additional acids which include: acetic, lactic, tartaric and citric which have a range of toxicities. This additive can be full of dangerous contaminants which form PFGA. Many fatty acids and their equivalents are produced using many levels of petroleum-based chemicals including: ether, tetrachloroethylene,

(which is considered to be a known carcinogen) and hexane. Extraction methods and filtering processes need to be revealed. The product is synthetic and used as a dough conditioner in yeast. Used in manufactured bakery products creating crusty breads as in rye bread, baked goods, biscuits, coffee whiteners, salad dressings, hot chocolate mixes, gravy granules, all types of dairy foods, edible fats, whipped fats, some meat products, and frozen pizza. Also used as an anti-splash agent in cooking oils and margarines. Is used as a protein builder in flours. Used as an emulsifier in mayonnaise and salad dressing and meat binder in sausages. As a by-product, meat (pork) cannot be excluded in the manufacturing of this product. May contribute to '*birth defects, cancer and genetic damage.*'[173] Also see: Dr Russell Blaylock, The Truth in Labelling.[174] On alert in the United States. Approved in the European Union, New Zealand and Australia. **Avoid**

| 472f **Avoid** | Mixed tartaric, acetic and fatty acid esters of glycerol or tartaric, acetic and fatty acid esters of glycerol (mixed) |
|---|---|

**Colour: Mixed acetic and tartaric acid esters[175] of mono and diglycerides[176] of fatty acids**
Mainly made from synthetic fats produced from plant origin but also from animal fats. Are used as emulsifiers. The fats are extracted using many levels of petroleum-based chemicals including: ether, hexane and tetrachloroethylene which are known carcinogens. Mainly used in vegetable oils. However, also used in cake mixes,

---

[173] http://thearticlebay.com
[174] www.truthinlabelling.org
[175] An organic compound made by replacing the hydrogen of an acid by an alkyl or other organic group.
[176] A glyceride consisting of two fatty acid chains.

oven-ready chips, baked goods, extensively used in all types of bread, dairy foods, margarine, ice cream and bakery products. Also used in high-fat bread, edible fats and meat products. In large amounts interferes with intestinal functions. May cause diarrhoea, thirst, dizziness and mental confusion. Also linked to: *'birth defects, cancer and genetic damage.'*[177] Check for approval in the United States, European Union, New Zealand and Australia. **Avoid**

| 473 **Avoid** | Sucrose esters of fatty acids |
|---|---|

**Colour: White to grey powder or gels of soft solids**
Esters[178] of sugar and fatty acids. Is a food emulsifier and stabiliser. The product is usually a mixture or ingredients that have been manufactured in the presence of solvents. Contains the ingredients: methyl alcohol and dimethyl formamide[179] also known as (methanamide). Methyl alcohol is usually called methanol and part of the hydroxyl group of chemicals. Dimethyl formamide is a common solvent for chemical reactions. Both are poison to the human system. The bought product may contain residues of solvents. Used in bakery goods including cakes and breads, dairy products, chewing gum, to stabilise margarine, mayonnaise, soups, desserts, and soft drinks. Although vegetable oils are used, animal by-products cannot be ruled out. May be used to stop fruit from spoiling by slowing the ripening process. May cause stomach pain, bloating, nausea, diarrhoea and is linked to poisoning. Approved in the United States, European Union, New Zealand and Australia. **Avoid**

---

[177] http://thearticlebay.com

[178] A chemical compound derived from an acid (organic or inorganic).

[179] Is highly corrosive, can cause excessive burning of the skin and eyes, and can cause death if it is ingested. Wise geek

| 475 Caution or Avoid | Polyglycerol esters of fatty acids |
|---|---|

**Colour: Light yellow to amber oil**
A group of poorly tested food additives. They are synthetic fatty acids that may be made from genetically modified soy-based raw material, rapeseed and maize. Used as a food emulsifier and stabiliser in cakes, margarines, milk, some dairy products, sponge cakes, breads, dietary products, sweets, lollies, ice cream, noodles, meats, shortening, confectionary and imitation cream products. Also used as an anti-foaming agent during the production or caramel colour which is used in many fizzy drinks, mainly colas and other like drinks. Also used in the pharmaceutical industry. They may contribute to health concerns or problems. Approved in the United States, European Union and New Zealand. Not approved in Australia. Caution or Avoid

| 476 Avoid | Polyglycerol esters of interesterified ricinoleic acid (PGPR) |
|---|---|

**Colour: Yellowish viscous liquid**
PGPR is an emulsifier extracted from castor or soy bean oil. Castor oil seed is also used to make the poison 'ricin'. Is a synthetic product including acetone-benzene. Is a petroleum solution used in the additive extraction, please also see 210. Can also be washed with potassium hydroxide. Is used in cheaper chocolate products to allow flow and decrease yield stress between molten chocolate, sugar and milk. Is used as a chocolate coating in: spreads, cocoa butter, spreadable fats, creamers, food dressings and commercially baked products. From a technical application PGPR is a plastic product. Polyglycerol is used in polymer coatings, paints; the manufacture of soaps,

coating for plastics and as an anti-fogging agent. There is a link between hyperactivity in children. Due to the castor oil content, there are concerns over embryo formation and miscarriage possibilities. Ingestion may cause gastrointestinal irritation, nausea, vomiting and diarrhoea. *'Linked to liver enlargement, kidney enlargement and severe allergic reactions.'*[180] On alert in the United States. Approved in the European Union. Approved in New Zealand and Australia. **Avoid**

| 477<br>**Avoid** | Propylene glycol mono-<br>and di-esters or<br>Propylene glycol esters<br>of fatty acids |
|---|---|

**Colour: White to cream waxy solid**
Is a synthetic compound manufactured from a mixture of propanediol[181] and natural fats. Can be derived from petroleum. Normal fats consists of glycerol and fatty acids, in this product, glycerol is replaced by propanediol an extract of corn syrup. The extraction of corn syrup needs identification. May be of animal or vegetable origin. Found in bakery products and puddings, confectionary, soft and fizzy drinks, ice cream, toppings, processed meats. Used in cosmetics and personal care products. May cause a *'reduction in the central nervous system, severe allergic reactions, renal changes and delayed growth.'*[182] Concentrations of propylene glycol may cause eczema and related allergies. On alert in the United States. Approved in the European Union. Approved in New Zealand and Australia. **Avoid**

---

[180] http://thearticlebay.com
[181] A solvent used in anti-freeze and brake fluid. Can be harmful if absorbed through the skin.
[182] http://thearticlebay.com

| 480 **Avoid** | Dioctyl sodium sulphosuccinate |
|---|---|

**Colour: White wax-like plastic solid**
Is produced by a reaction of octane with malic acid and a combination of propanediol (which can be derived from petroleum) and natural fats. Is used as an emulsifier, dispersant and wetting agent in pesticide preparations. Helps syrups to evenly spread through dairy products, is used in edible gums, soft drinks, cordials, and syrups. The substance is at toxic levels in some rainbow trout. May aggravate food intolerance in infants and children and those people sensitive to sulphur added products. May cause cramps and abdominal pain. Will irritate eyes, lungs and skin. Product is currently under research and investigation. Assists in putting out fires and in controlling ocean oil spillage. Approved in the United States. On alert in the European Union. Approved in New Zealand and Australia. **Avoid**

| 481 **Caution** or **Avoid** | Sodium lactylate (i) Sodium stearoyl lactylate (ii) Sodium oleyl lactylate (SSL) |
|---|---|

**Colour: Yellowish powder or brittle solid**
Is a neutralised food grade soda ash (sodium carbonate) or caustic soda (concentrated sodium hydroxide) additive. Is used as an emulsifier and stabiliser in flour products and many commercially produced foods. Also used to improve texture in baked goods, breads and dough; is also used as a dough conditioner. Used in pancakes, waffles, cereals, pastas, instant rice, desserts, icings, fillings, sugar confectionary, sweets, lollies, beverage mixes, dehydrated potatoes, chewing gum, dietetic foods, snacks, dips,

sauces, minced and diced canned meats. Also added to whipped vegetables, oil toppings, icings, desserts, whipping agents, salad dressings, French salad dressing, soups, non-dairy creamers, cream liqueur drinks and pet food. Inadequate research on this additive found. In the United States, on alert (ii) sodium oleyl lactylate. In the European Union all additives are on alert. All are approved in New Zealand and Australia. **Caution** or **Avoid**

| 482<br>**Caution** or **Avoid** | Calcium lactylate<br>**(i) Calcium stearoyl lactylate**<br>**(i) Calcium oleyl lactylate** |
|---|---|

**Colour: White to yellowish brittle powder**
Is synthetic additive used as an emulsifier and stabiliser in flour and dough produced foods. This additive ensures a thin crust after baking. It lessens staling of breads and cake products also allows for a small pore structure in sponges, light cakes and food delicacies. Used in the production of fine bakery, various breads and cake mixtures, sweets and lollies, confectionary, oil emulsions, cereals and potato-based appetisers, canned or chopped mincemeat products, cream and cream mixtures, hot drink powders and breakfast cereals. In some people it may cause hives, bloating, skin rash, irritability, and irritable bowel syndrome (IBS), migraine, stomachache, nausea, headaches, runny nose or coughing. All additives are on alert in the United States. Calcium lactylate only approved in the European Union. All approved in New Zealand and Australia. **Caution** or **Avoid**

| 491 Caution or Avoid | Sorbitan monostearate |
|---|---|

**Colour: Light brown beads or flakes of waxy solid**
In commercial production, this product is synthetic. Used as an emulsifier, thickener and sweetener – is a modifying agent. The chemical origin of this additive cannot be determined; more research is needed. Is used in fine bakery, cakes, ice cream, flavoured milk, cake mixes, whipping cream, whipped vegetables, oil toppings, biscuit or cookie coatings, cream substitutes, coconut spread, beverages, protective coatings on fruits and vegetables, frozen puddings, candy, confectionary and sweets. Also used in icing. The toxicology for this product has not been researched or investigated. Is used in synthetic fibre machinery fluid and brighteners in the leather and tanning industry. Also used in pesticides and in various applications in the plastics industry. Is linked to *'eczema, intestinal disorder, kidney stones and severe allergic reactions.*[183] Approved in the United States, European Union, New Zealand and Australia. **Caution** or **Avoid**

| 492 Caution or Avoid | Sorbitan tristearate (STS) |
|---|---|

**Colour: Cream, wax like powder**
Is a synthetic and emulsifier, (which can increase the absorption of fat) within polysorbates. Is the esterification of sorbitol with synthetic stearic acid possibly derived from food fats or possibly palm oils. Is used as a dispersing agent in food and in aerosol sprays. Also used in fine bakery products and decoration. Used in baker's yeast, oil emulsions, milk and cream mixtures, marmalades, cocoa-

---

[183] http://thearticlebay.com

based candies and sweets, chocolates or chocolate compound, margarine, spreadable spreads, edible ices, desserts, dietary supplements, chewing gum, liquid mixtures of fruit and vegetables, sugar-based candies or lollies and food supplements. May include animal fat (pork). As 491, is linked to: *'eczema, intestinal disorders, kidney stones and severe allergic reaction.'* See EFSA[184] On alert in the United States. Approved in the European Union, New Zealand and Australia. **Caution** or **Avoid**

---

[184] https://fr-en.openfoodfacts.org

**Your Notes**

..................................................................

..................................................................

..................................................................

..................................................................

..................................................................

..................................................................

..................................................................

..................................................................

..................................................................

..................................................................

..................................................................

..................................................................

..................................................................

..................................................................

..................................................................

..................................................................

..................................................................

..................................................................

**Devils:** Mineral salts (often used as anti-caking agents (500 range)

| Devil Numbers | Additive |
|---|---|
| **500**<br>Caution or Avoid | **Sodium bicarbonate**<br>**(i) Sodium carbonate**<br>**(ii) Sodium hydrogen carbonate**<br>**(iii) Sodium sesquicarbonate** |

**Colour: White solid crystalline powder**
Used in food mainly as a raising agent. In mass production can be a synthetic product. Synthetic products are developed through the use of electrolysis and sea water with the Solvay process[185]. Used in soft and fizzy drinks, beer making, expansion of batter, texture and grain in pancakes, cakes, soda bread and many baked foods. Large amounts can cause deterioration of the gut, gastric conditions and poor circulation. For further reading please see footnote below.[186] On alert in the United States (ii). On alert in the European Union (ii) and (iii). On alert in New Zealand and Australia (ii) and (iii). Caution or Avoid

| | |
|---|---|
| **501**<br>Caution | **Potassium bicarbonate**<br>**Potassium carbonate**<br>**(i) (ii)** |

**Colour: colourless, odourless, slightly salty substance**
From the mineral called Kalicinite which is rarely found in its natural form. In commercial use is produced by reacting

---

[185] The industrial process using ammonia-soda in the production of sodium carbonate.
[186] https://medsafe.govt.nz

potassium carbonate liquid with carbon dioxide, then re-crystallizing the product. Is used in cocoa, confectionary, custard powder and other food products. Also used in the pharmaceutical industry. If inhaled will irritate the lungs. Approved in the United States, potassium carbonates and potassium carbonate (i). On alert in the United States potassium (ii). Approved in the European Union potassium carbonates and potassium carbonate (i). Approved in New Zealand and Australia, potassium carbonates and potassium carbonate (i) and on alert potassium carbonate (ii). **Caution**

| 503 Avoid | Ammonium carbonates (i) Ammonium carbonate (ii) Ammonium hydrogen carbonate |
|---|---|

**Colour: White crystalline solid**

Is produced from calcium carbonate and ammonium sulphate. Is used as an adjusting acidity regulator and modifying mineral salt. Used in baked products, baking powder, cocoa products, many forms of confectionary, sweets, lollies, ice cream and related food products. Also used in some medications. Can alter the pH balance of urine and may cause irritation to mucous membranes and the stomach lining. Can also cause the loss of calcium and magnesium from the human body. Is linked to: '*nerve cell destruction, neurological disorders, is a neurotoxin and severe allergic reactions.*'[187] Ammonium carbonate and ammonium carbonate (i) approved in the United States, ammonium hydrogen carbonate (ii) on alert. Ammonium carbonate and ammonium carbonate (i) approved in the European Union, ammonium hydrogen carbonate (ii) on alert. On alert in New Zealand and Australia ammonium carbonate (i). Ammonium carbonates and ammonium hydrogen carbonate (ii) approved in New Zealand and Australia. **Avoid**

---

[187] http://thearticlebay.com

| 504<br>Safe or Caution | Magnesium carbonate<br>(i) Magnesium carbonate<br>(ii) Magnesium hydroxide carbonate |
| --- | --- |

**Colour: White inorganic solid salt**

Is produced from magnesium hydroxide but occurs as a natural mineral. Is an anti-caking, bleaching, adjusting and modifying agent. Is used in granular foods, sugar, dry mixes, icing sugar and salt. Is a low-sodium salt substitute. In moderation, is a valuable mineral for the human system. Approved in the United States, European Union, New Zealand and Australia. Safe or Caution

| 507<br>Avoid | Hydrochloric acid<br>HCI |
| --- | --- |

**Colour: Colourless inorganic chemical**

Is a highly corrosive compound manufactured commercially from sulphuric acid and sodium chloride; alternatively through a reaction of hydrogen and chlorine gases. Is an inorganic chemical system used in food production, food enhancement, food ingredients, food additives and as an acidity regulator. Used in fructose, citric acid, cold sore treatments, hydrolysed vegetable proteins, gelatine, corn flour and the malting of beer. Also used in textile production, chloride, fertilizer, dye and rubber production, artificial pigments for paints. Used in the creation of PVC and in the production of formaldehyde. Is corrosive to mucus membranes, will cause chest pains, inflammation and coughing. Is corrosive to the mouth and stomach. Can also cause haemorrhage, gastric ulceration, intestinal irritation, perforation, nausea and vomiting. May be carcinogenic when mixed with formaldehyde. Approved in the United States, European Union, New Zealand and Australia. Avoid

| 508<br>Avoid | Potassium chloride<br>KCL |
|---|---|

**Colour: White colourless to white to shades of yellow crystal**

Is extracted from the minerals sylvite, carnallite and potash from many areas globally. In the process of manufacturing chlorine, mercury is used to create an amalgam with sodium. After polonium, mercury is considered to be an extreme poison and can be deadly when used for human consumption. Is used as a food enrichment additive. Also used in drinking water, brewing beer and other fermented alcohols, many bread varieties, salt substitutes, gelling agents, flavouring agents, flavour enhancers, nutrient supplement, pH control agent and stabiliser. Also used in reduced sodium foods, potato crisps and chips. Other than normal intake can cause irregular heartbeat, stomach pain, muscle weakness, diarrhoea, vomiting or nausea, gastric ulceration, numbness, tingling in the hands, feet and mouth. Allergic reaction signs are: hives, itching, trouble breathing, swelling in the mouth, face lips, throat and tongue, hoarseness in the voice, red, swollen and blistered skin outbreaks. Is linked to: irritating and stomach discomfort, haemorrhage, chest pain or pressure, signs of bowel problems: black, sticky or bloody stools, mucus in the stools, pain and constipation. Approved in the United State, European Union, New Zealand and Australia. Avoid

| 509<br>Caution or Avoid | Calcium chloride |
|---|---|

**Colour: An inorganic white chemical compound**

Is an ionic mineral compound containing calcium, chlorine and in some instances aluminium. In the process of manufacturing, mercury is used to create an amalgam with sodium. Possibly synthetic when produced by the Solvay process[188]. Used as a firming agent in chocolate manufacturing for the global marketplace and as a salt substitute. Also used in brewing beer and other fermented alcohols. Used in jelly manufacture and in many varieties of breads, Turkish delight and like confectionary, potato chips or crisps and as a gelling agent. Also used in tofu and in a wide range of cheese manufacturing, canned fruit and vegetables and the pickling industry. Other applications: aquarium water stabilisation, ice and dust control on roads, used in cement in the building industry and for brine in refrigeration. Will cause intestinal ulceration, intestinal problems, haemorrhage, nausea and vomiting. Approved in the United States, European Union, New Zealand and Australia. **Caution** or **Avoid**

| 510<br>**Caution** or **Avoid** | Ammonium chloride |
|---|---|

**Colour: White crystalline salt**
A product derived from hydrochloric acid and ammonia. Used as a bulking and improving agent in manufactured and commercial food production. Is used in flour-based products including bread and bread mixes, and as a low-sodium salt substitute in many foods. Used as a nutritive media for yeast. Also used in cough medicines and medications. Is also used as a compound fertiliser in the growing of: wheat, rice, barley, sugarcane and palm. Used in textile printing, bonding plywood and as an additive in cleaning products. Should be avoided if you suffer with impaired kidney or liver functions. Approved in the United States. On alert in the European Union. Approved in New Zealand and Australia. **Caution** or **Avoid**

---

[188] An industrial process for obtaining sodium carbonate from limestone, ammonia, and brine.

| 511 | Magnesium chloride |
|---|---|
| **Avoid** | |

**Colour: White powder produced from sea water**
In its natural form, is a natural mineral produced by the sea and oceans' evaporation. Is also found in natural green leafy vegetables, meat, and some fish. The commercially manufactured product also uses sea water or brine however, in the process of production chlorine and mercury are used to create an amalgam with sodium. Depending on production methods, can contain aluminium. Is used to purify drinking water, also used as a bulking, firming agent in many foods. Used in tofu, baby formulas, meats, cereals, snack foods: chips and crisps, soups, sauces, frozen entrees, snack bars, sports and electrolyte drinks. Is dangerous for people suffering from kidney disease. Is linked to: '*endocrine disruption; is a neurotoxin and linked to cancer.*'[189] Can cause a toxic reaction in some people. Approved in the United States, European Union, New Zealand and Australia. **Avoid**

| 512 | Stannous chloride |
|---|---|
| **Avoid** | |

**Colour: A white crystalline solid**
Is prepared from hydrochloric acid[190] (spirits of salt) and tin ores. Is used in many canned or tinned foods including baby and infant formula, baby and follow-up formulas, canned baby foods, canned beans and asparagus, dietary foods and foods with medical purposes. Causes headaches, skin and mucous irritation also nausea, negative effects to

---

[189] http://thearticlebay.com
[190] A strong corrosive acid used in industry.

the central nervous system resulting in cardiac arrhythmia and paralysis. Exposure may result in death. Can also irritate eyes and skin. Is used in the production of polyvinylchloride for plastics. Approved in the United States, European Union, New Zealand and Australia. **Avoid**

| 514 **Avoid** | Sodium sulphates<br>(i) Sodium sulfate<br>(ii) Sodium hydrogen sulphate or<br>Sulphate of soda |
|---|---|
| **Colour: White inorganic crystal**<br>In commercial production is prepared from salt and sulphuric acid. Some natural products are mined. Is used as an anti-caking agent and for diluting colour powders in biscuits, chewing gum, beer, sweets, lollies and confectionary. May upset the human body's water balance. Also used in detergents and paper making. Dangerous for people suffering from liver and heart disorders. May cause eye and skin irritation. May affect those adults and children who suffer with asthma. Due to the high salt content, not recommended for infants, young children, pregnant women or lactating mothers. On alert in the United States (ii) Sodium hydrogen sulphate. Approved in the European Union, New Zealand and Australia. **Avoid** ||

| 515 **Avoid** | Potassium sulphates<br>SOP<br>(i) Potassium sulphate<br>(ii) Potassium hydrogen sulfate |
|---|---|
| **Colour: White or cream crystalline salt**<br>Prepared from potassium chloride and sulphuric acid. Used as an anti-caking agent for diluting colour powders in beer, biscuits, a wide range of confectionary and chewing gum. ||

Is linked to intestinal bleeding and kidney enlargement. The dust from potassium sulphate can upset the human body's water balance. Can also cause asthma and eye irritation. Is classified as hazardous. Approved in the United States: potassium hydrogen sulphate, (ii) on alert. Approved in the European Union: potassium hydrogen sulphate, (ii) on alert. Approved in New Zealand and Australia: potassium hydrogen sulphate, (ii) on alert. **Avoid**

| 516 **Avoid** | Calcium sulphate Also know as: Plaster of Paris Gypsum and Drierite |
|---|---|

**Colour: Crystals solid or powdered solid**
Is an inorganic compound and mineral salt derived from limestone (gypsum). Used as a sequestrant,[191] buffer, firming and stabilizing agent. Used as a coagulant in many food products including: tofu, soy products, some cheeses, frozen desserts, jelly and jelly-based foods also used in a wide range of flours, bakery products and as a bleaching agent for bread-based foods. Used in a wide array of preserves, vegetable condiments, tomato condiments and sauces, sweets, candies and confectionary. Also used in artificial sweeteners, dried eggs and toothpaste. Absorbs the body's moisture, will harden quickly as in plaster of Paris. May cause intestinal blockage or constipation. Can cause gastrointestinal discomfort, liver poisoning; can affect the human nervous and respiratory systems. Approved in the United States and in the European Union. On alert in New Zealand and Australia. **Avoid**

---

[191] Forms a shell (chelate complexes) with polyvalent metal ions especially copper, iron and nickel, which can prevent oxidation of the fats in food.

| 518 **Avoid** | Magnesium sulphate |
|---|---|

**Colour: Colourless or white, granular, crystalline powder**

Is prepared from magnesium salts and sulphuric acid. Is used as a firming agent for medications in the pharmaceutical industry also in laxative treatments. Is also used in food supplements and as a mineral in infant formulas. Used in beer and related drinks. Can be hazardous to people with kidney or with related problems. May cause congenital anomalies or birth defects. Is linked to cancer. Approved in the United States. Not approved in the European Union. Approved in New Zealand and Australia. **Avoid**

| 519 **Avoid** | Copper II (Cupric sulphate) Also known as: (Blue vitriol and bluestone) |
|---|---|

**Colour: Blue stone solid crystal**

Is a mineral salt produced industrially by treating copper metal with hot concentrated sulphuric acid or oxides with diluted sulphuric acid. Is used as a preservative and anti-caking agent. Also helps food to retain and intensify its colour. As a preservative, helps against food deterioration caused by micro-organisms. Is a cumulative poison. Used in meat products and cereals. Is also used in infant formula as a mineral supplement. (Should not be taken separately). Is linked to gastrointestinal problems. Is a neurotoxin. People suffering with kidney or liver problems should avoid. On alert in the United States. On alert in the European Union. Is approved in New Zealand and Australia. **Avoid**

| 520 Avoid | Aluminium sulphate (anhydrous) |
|-----------|--------------------------------|

**Colour: Is an odourless white or off-white crystalline solid or powder**

Is manufactured by combining aluminium hydroxide and sulphuric acid. Used as a firming agent and starch in the food industry. Is found in manufactured beer, commercially made proteins and pickled vegetables. Is added to tap and drinking water, also added to antacid medications. Evidence is showing that the accumulation of aluminium is toxic and linked to Parkinson-type diseases. High accumulated levels of neurofibrillary tangles and neuritic plaques are found in the human brain cells of Alzheimer's patients. Studies have not revealed whether the aluminium accumulation is causative or resultant of the disease. May contribute to liver, disease, premature senility, osteoporosis and toxicity of the nervous system. Aluminium inhibits the uptake of B-vitamins. Used in the construction and aerospace industries. Also used in foil and aerosol cans. See 173, http://thearticlebay.com. On alert in the United States. Approved in the European Union. On alert in New Zealand and Australia. **Avoid**

| 521 Avoid | Sodium aluminium sulphate (Soda alum or sodium alum) |
|-----------|------------------------------------------------------|

**Colour: Fine white powder**

Is manufactured using sodium and aluminium sulphates. Used as an acidity regulator, bleaching agent and firming agent. Is used in flour and flour products, many varieties of cheeses and in a wide range of confectionary, sweets, candies and lollies. It strengthens vegetable products while in processing. Also used in the production of baking powder. Aluminium hinders the uptake of B-vitamin from a balanced diet. Can interfere with liver function and premature senility. Aluminium is linked to: '*Alzheimer's disease, dementia and Parkinson's, osteoporosis, toxicity of the nervous system and kidney disease.*'[192] Contained in antacid tablets, antiperspirants, and aluminium pots. See 173, http://thearticlebay.com. On alert in the United States. Approved in the European Union. On alert in New Zealand and Australia. **Avoid**

| 522 **Avoid** | Potassium aluminium sulphate |
|---|---|

**Colour: large transparent crystalline fragments or crystals**

Is manufactured from potassium and aluminium sulphates. Is used as an acidity regulator and widely used in baking powder. Is extensively used in the food industry in flour and flour-based products including: breads, cakes and rolls. Also used as a bleaching agent and the stabilisation of colour in flour. Used in many varieties of cheeses, confectionary including sweets, lollies and candies. Also used in the building and construction industries and in the aerospace industry. Is used as a base in many antiperspirants or deodorants. Evidence shows that toxic aluminium accumulates in body cells, which links it to many illnesses, including Parkinson and associated diseases. Also identified, the accumulation of aluminium contributing to neurofibrillary tangles and neuritic plaques in Alzheimer patients. It's not known whether the outcome is a resultant role or causative. Aluminium will block the uptake of B-vitamins from food or health supplements. See 173, http://thearticlebay.com. On alert in the United States. Approved in the European Union. Not approved in New Zealand or Australia. **Avoid**

---

[192] http://thearticlebay.com

| 523 | Aluminium ferric ammonium sulphate |
|:---:|:---:|

**Colour: White crystalline double sulphate**
Prepared from natural aluminium sulphate. Ferric sulphate is mixed with ammonium sulphate and crystallized to achieve ammonium iron (iii). Is used as an acid source and regulator in baking powder in industrial and commercial bakeries. Stabilises colour in food products. Is used as a firming and stabilising agent. Is linked to: *'premature senility, Alzheimer's disease, dementia and Parkinson's disease, osteoporosis, toxicity to the nervous system; danger for people with kidney disease.'*[193] Out of date, unsold aluminium cans containing soft drink may contain higher levels of aluminium than newly produced cans. Most deodorants and antiperspirants contain levels of aluminium that stop perspiration but also stop the body discharging toxins through sweating. See 173, http://thearticlebay.com.On alert in the United States. Approved in the European Union. On alert and not allowed in New Zealand and Australia. **Avoid**

| 524 **Avoid** | Aluminium ferric ammonium sulphate, Aluminium-ammonium |
|:---:|:---:|

**Colour: White solid ionic compound**
Sodium hydroxide is highly toxic and corrosive. Is prepared from natural salt (sodium carbonate), mixed with lime to form an alkali. Is used in the manufacture of soaps and corrosive caustic soda. Is also used in drain cleaners and other cleaning agents. Also used as an acidity regulator in many food products. Is used in baking soda, sour cream, jams, cocoa products, tinned vegetables, some edible fats and oils. Also used to produce the glaze on pretzels, in the

---

[193] http://thearticlebay.com

production of caramel and to blacken olives. Can cause severe burns. If ingested, can cause diarrhoea, stomach pain, allergies, adverse reactions, shock and death. Banned in some countries. Approved in the United States and the European Union. On alert and not permitted in New Zealand and Australia. **Avoid**

| 525 Avoid | Potassium hydroxide Potassium lye or Caustic potash |
|---|---|

**Colour: Whit to nearly white flakes, sicks or pellets**
Is a mineral toxic, highly corrosive, caustic salt and chemical used as an acidity regulator in some food production. Is used in cocoa and cocoa manufactured food products, cheeses and cheese products, jams and conserves and to blacken black olives. Causes burning in the mouth and throat, stomach swelling, swelling of the stomach lining and membranes, vomiting, pain and shock. Is used in the manufacture of soap and bleaching and as a paint remover. Approved in the United States and the European Union. On alert in New Zealand or Australia. **Avoid**

| 526 Avoid | Calcium hydroxide |
|---|---|

**Colour: Colourless white crystal**
Is a product of lime used in the food industry as a firming and neutralising agent and as an acidity regulator in the production of wine. Also used in beer making, the glaze on pretzels, cocoa products, edible fats and oils, jams, sour cream, tinned vegetables. Also used to regulate acidity in frozen food products and the preservation of eggs. Can

give severe allergic reactions, is highly corrosive and toxic. High intake contributes to tissue damage, rupture of blood cells, the development of kidney stones, heart arrhythmia and possible cardiac arrest. Approved in the United States, European Union, New Zealand and Australia. **Avoid**

| 529<br>**Caution** or **Avoid** | Calcium oxide<br>(Quick lime) |
|---|---|

**Colour: White, crystalline,** caustic, alkaline solid
A mineral salt prepared from chalk. Used to remove impurities and as an improving, modifying agent in many food products which include: yeast for nutrient in many types of breads and bakery goods, confectionary, tinned peas, sour cream, dairy products and sugar. Used in the preparation of intestines for sausages. Contributes to severe allergic reactions, is highly corrosive and toxic. May be safe in small quantities. Reacts in water, can cause burns to eyes and skin. Approved in the United States, European Union, New Zealand and Australia. **Caution** or **Avoid**

| 530<br>**Avoid** | Magnesium oxide |
|---|---|

**Colour: White solid hygroscopic[194] mineral**
Is produced by the calcinations of magnesium hydroxide or magnesium carbonate. Also used in soil and groundwater remediation, drinking water, wastewater, waste treatment industries and in air emissions treatment. Used in the food industry as an anti-caking agent. Is added

---

[194] Draws moisture from the air.

to canned peas, cocoa and their related products, frozen dairy products, butter and used in the pharmaceutical industry in medications. Causes itching, rashes, weakness, tiredness, vomiting, mood swings and numbness. *'Is non-chelated, so it doesn't absorb well...'*[195] This product does not chemically bind to the body's amino acids. Banned in some countries.

Approved in the United States and the European Union. Not approved in New Zealand and Australia. **Avoid**

| 535<br>**Avoid** | **Sodium ferrocyanide<br>Also known as<br>(Yellow prussiate of<br>soda)** |
|---|---|

**Colour: Is a yellow crystalline solid**
Is produced industrially from hydrogen cyanide, calcium hydroxide and ferrous chloride. This anti-caking agent contains cyanide and is often added to food grade salt or table salt to stop sticking and to maintain flow. Can be toxic combined with acid. Read the label. Large doses can harm the human body. Used in industry, in photography, gold plating and galvanising silver and pewter. Approved in the United States, European Union, New Zealand and Australia. **Avoid**

| 536<br>**Avoid** | **Potassium ferrocyanide<br>(Yellow prussiate of<br>potash)** |
|---|---|

**Colour: Lemon to yellow crystal**
Is a by-product of coal and gas production. A synthetic crystal manufactured from hydrogen ferrocyanide and potassium hydroxide. Contains cyanide. Is used as an anti-

---

[195]https://www.newsmax.com Jen Krausz 06/05/2016

caking agent in the removal of metal in wine, seasonings and spices. May be included in salt substitutes, read the label. Reduces transportation of oxygen to the blood. Causes breathing difficulties, headaches, dizziness and feeling unwell. Can cause problems for asthmatics and produce allergic reactions. On alert in the United States. Approved in the European Union, New Zealand and Australia. **Avoid**

| 537 <br> **Avoid** | Ferrous <br> hexacyanomanganate |
|---|---|

**Colour: May resemble a black liquorice powder derived from salmiak**
Is manufactured from mangano-cyanide, iron hydroxide and hydroxide. Is used as an anti-caking agent. Also used in the manufacture of many liquorice flavoured sweets, lollies and candies. On alert in the United States. Not permitted in the European Union, New Zealand and Australia. **Avoid**

| 538 <br> **Avoid** | Calcium ferrocyanide |
|---|---|

**Colour: Yellow or crystalline powder**
Is a synthetic crystallising agent. Is manufactured from ferrocyanide, hydrogen and calcium hydroxide. Used as a salt substitute, anti-caking and food improvement agent. Is used in seasonings and spices. Also used in the removal of metal from wine. Will harm the human body causing dizziness, difficulties in breathing, headaches and can reduce oxygen movement in the blood. Animal studies have proven kidney damage, skin and eye irritation. On

alert in the United States. Approved in the European Union. On alert in New Zealand and Australia. **Avoid**

| 539 Avoid | Sodium thiosulphate |
|---|---|

**Colour: Colourless crystalline compound**
Is an inorganic compound produced from the liquid waste products of sodium sulphide or sulphur dyeing and manufacture. Is used as a sequestrant and anti-oxidant to prevent the browning process of many manufactured potato products. Is used in water treatment, photography, print development and medicine. Approved in the United States. On alert in the European Union, New Zealand and Australia. **Avoid**

| 540 Avoid | Dicalcium diphosphate or (Acid calcium phosphate) |
|---|---|

**Colour: White powder**
Is an inorganic compound from one of the sodium phosphates. Is used as an emulsifier in a variety of different manufactured foods. Is used as a popular food additive in dietary, calcium supplements. Also used in breakfast cereals and condensed milk. Used to enrich flour and powdered products. Used as an additive to noodles, in dog foods and dog treats and in tablet manufacture in the pharmaceutical industry. Used in poultry feed and toothpaste. See additive 450. May be adverse reactions. Can lead to osteoporosis and other like diseases. Check for approval in the United States, European Union and New Zealand. Banned in Australia. **Avoid**

| 541<br>Avoid | Sodium aluminium phosphates<br>(i) Sodium aluminium phosphate, acidic<br>(ii) Sodium aluminium phosphate, basic |
|---|---|

**Colour: White odourless powder**

A synthetic food additive produced from sodium hydroxide, aluminium and phosphoric acid. May contain cyanide. Is used as an acidity regulator, emulsifier and bleaching agent in flour and flour produced goods. Also used in baking powder. Is contained in commercially produced food including: baked foods, cheeses and cheese products, many forms of confectionary, sweets, lollies and candies. Can be an ingredient of commercially made mincemeat products, stews, frozen fish and frozen fish products. Is added to tap water. Not suitable for babies or people suffering from heart or kidney problems. Aluminium is toxic and accumulates in the human body. Limits the uptake of the B-vitamins from naturally produced food. Widely available in antacid medications. Is linked to Parkinson's and Parkinson-type diseases including Alzheimer's disease. *'There is evidence to suggest that the accumulation of aluminium in the cells of the nervous system could be toxic. It is found in abnormally high levels in the brain cells of Alzheimer's disease sufferers, accumulated in the neurofibrillary tangles and neuritic plaques...'*[196] May cause skeletal deformations. Pregnant women and lactating mothers should avoid. Approved in the United States and European Union. Approved in New Zealand and Australia sodium aluminium phosphates and sodium aluminium basic. On alert (i) **Avoid**

---

[196] http://www.wotzinurfood.com

| 542 Caution or Avoid | Bone phosphate |
|---|---|

**Colour: Whit to pale cream odourless powder**
Is a product manufactured from the steaming and degreased bones of pigs and cattle. Is used as an anti-caking agent and emulsifier in dried milk for coffee machines, in food supplements; a filler for tablets, and in cane sugar. More research is needed and required for this product. On alert in the United States and the European Union. Approved in the New Zealand and Australia. Caution or Avoid

| 551 Safe or Caution | Silicon dioxide, amorphous (Silica) |
|---|---|

**Colour: White amorphous powder, beads or granules**
Derived from sand (silica) and used in many food products. Silica is important to maintain health and wellbeing. *'If used as an anti-caking agent to food product it is not safe when the Si02 quantity is more than 2 percent of the food's weight. It should be made by a process known as vapour phase hydrolysis. If it is manufactured by any other process, then the recommended particle size of Si02 should not exceed the safety norms.'*[197] Is added to thickeners and stabilisers in beer, confectionary, dried milk, sausages and sweeteners. Is dangerous if inhaled. Approved in the United States, European Union, New Zealand and Australia. Safe or Caution

---

[197] http://www.wotzinurfood.com

| 552 Safe or Caution | Calcium silicate |
|---|---|

**Colour: Fine white to off-white powder**

May also be manufactured as a synthetic. Check ingredients. Is derived from limestone, silicified skeletons of single-cell plankton, chalk and selected sand. Is produced from calcium silicate, hydrochloric acid and sodium silicate. (Burnt lime is treated with hydrochloric acid to produce calcium chloride). When the calcium silicate is precipitated out, the solution is then treated with clear sodium silicate. Used as an anti-caking, anti-clumping agent. Is used in salt, dried eggs, baking powder, egg yolks, grated cheese, egg whites, antacids, as a dusting agent on chewing gum and as a coating agent on rice. Is used to melt ice on roads. Further research needed on the manufacturing or extraction processes. Generally assumed as safe for human consumption. Is approved in the United States, European Union, New Zealand and Australia. Safe or Caution

| 553 Avoid | (i) Magnesium silicate (ii) Magnesium trisilicate (iii) talc |
|---|---|

**Colour: Fine white odourless powder**

Magnesium silicate is a synthetic additive. Is derived from asbestos, magnesium sulphate, sepiolite[198], steatite[199] and sodium silicate. Is used as an anti-caking agent, filling agent and coating agent. Is used as a dusting agent on rice and is linked to the world's highest number of people with

---

[198] Light porous clay derived from cuttlefish.
[199] Soapstone

stomach cancer. Is used in and on chewing gum often listed under the name (gum base). Also used in chocolate of many brands, confectionary, sweets, lollies and in glazes used on many foods. Is used as a filling agent in antacid tablets and medical tablet manufacture. Is used in the manufacture of rubber as a filler, as a bleaching agent in many products. Also used to correct odour in sanitary pads, condoms and possibly baby and toddler disposable nappies. Used in baby talcum and adult talcum powders. Check the manufacturers' labels. Is used in the manufacture of paints and resins. May be linked to lung cancer, kidney disease and damage also severe allergic reactions. A dangerous additive. Banned in some countries. Approved in the United States. On alert in the United States (ii) magnesium trisilicate. Approved in the European Union. Approved in New Zealand and Australia. **Avoid**

| 554 **Avoid** | Sodium aluminosilicaate |
|---|---|

**Colour: Fine white, odourless amorphous powder or bead**
Is a synthetic unstructured, neurotoxic food additive used widely in the global food industry. Can be dangerous as it contains aluminium. Is used as an anti-caking agent in a range of flours and bakery products, egg mixes, sugar and sugar products. Also used in salt and in dried milk substitutes. Aluminium is a neurotoxin and linked to Alzheimer's disease. Aluminium causes many illnesses to the human body including: *'premature senility, Parkinson's disease, osteoporosis, toxicity of and to the nervous systems and can be dangerous to people suffering with kidney disease.'*[200] Aluminium is also linked to mental

---

[200] http://thearticlebay.com

315

health problems, general poor negative health, headaches, rheumatism and the general feelings of ill health. Also used in deodorants and antiperspirant. Approved in the United States, European Union, New Zealand and Australia. **Avoid**

| 555 **Avoid** | Potassium aluminium silicate |
|---|---|

**Colour: Colourless, white flowing powder or needles**
Produced from many minerals including silicon, potassium and aluminium. Aluminium is a neurotoxic and extremely toxic to the human body. Is used as an anti-caking agent in many food products including: dried milk and dried milk substitutes, sugar products and food goods made from sugar, egg mixes and a range of flours. Is linked to many illnesses and diseases including: Alzheimer's, Parkinson's, which may be directly linked to aluminium, Osteoporosis, many forms of kidney disease, premature senility, bone loss, stomach problems, heart conditions, mental illness, rheumatism, bowel conditions and headaches. Aluminium is also absorbed through the body when using deodorants. May also be ingested through the use of aluminium pots for cooking, antacid medications and aluminium foil. Approved in the United States, European Union, New Zealand and Australia. **Avoid**

| 556 **Avoid** | Calcium aluminium silicate |
|---|---|

**Colour: White, fine free-flowing powder**
Is manufactured from many different minerals. Also contains aluminium, a dangerous and toxic metal harmful to the human body. Aluminium is a neurotoxic which is found in many manufactured food products. Is used as an anti-caking agent, sequestrant, firming and raising agent. Used in many dried milk powders and milk substitutes. Also used in egg mixes, cheeses, pre-prepared vegetable foods, flours and pasta. Has been linked to Alzheimer's and Parkinson's type diseases. Is known to cause placental problems during pregnancy, causes bone loss, stomach problems, bowel and kidney problems, heart conditions, rheumatism, mental health conditions, headaches, and the general feeling of being unwell. Is known to cause adverse reactions and severe allergies. Approved in the United States, European Union, New Zealand and Australia. **Avoid**

| 558 **Safe** or **Caution** | Bentonite |
|---|---|

**Colour: Grey, beige, green colour**
Is found in impure clay. Bentonite is an absorbent aluminium which means, in moderation, it can be ingested and digested by the human gut. Is used as an anti-caking agent. Used in the pharmaceutical industry for external skin preparations. Also used in the manufactured food industry in edible fats, oils, wine and sugar. May be added to manufactured food products. Can be used in marshmallows. To increase detoxification is used in Natto soybean breakfast foods. Helps in the removal of

albicans[201] and Candida. Approved in the United States, European Union, New Zealand and Australia. Safe or Caution

| 559 Avoid | Aluminium silicate (Kaolin) |
|---|---|

**Colour: White clay formed by weathering of aluminium minerals**
Produced from aluminium oxide and silicone dioxide to produce an aluminosilicate fibrous material. Used as a mineral salt and anti-caking agent also used to carry food aromas when cooking. Is used in dried milk in coffee machines. Is known to be linked to Alzheimer's and Parkinson's diseases. Also causes heart conditions, mental health problems, rheumatism, headaches, bone loss, stomach conditions and discomfort, kidney, bowel problems and contributes to a number of diseases. Aluminium can cause intestinal obstruction and tumours. On alert in the United States. Approved in the European Union, New Zealand and Australia. Avoid

| 560 Avoid | Potassium silicate |
|---|---|

**Colour: Solid, glassy lump**
Is used as an anti-caking agent. Is synthesized by treating silica with potassium. Is used in welding, electrode plating and in glass for acid resistance. Found acute toxicity when testing fish, invertebrates and algae. On alert in the United

---

[201] A common pathogenic member of the human gut flora.

States and the European Union. Approved in New Zealand and Australia. **Avoid**

| 570 <br> **Avoid** <br> | **Stearic acid or Fatty acid** |
|---|---|

**Colour: White flake or white powder**
Found in natural animal fats and un-tampered vegetable oils. In mass production, is synthesized and used as an anti-caking agent and food additive. May be genetically modified. Can be made from soybean, rapeseed and maize. However, in mass production is usually made from highly toxic cottonseed oil. Cottonseed is grown as an industrial crop and is not meant for the food supply market, therefore, it can be sprayed with highly dangerous pesticides and toxins. Pesticides concentrate in the soil, thus entering the food chain via the plant. Is used as a filler in dietary supplements and the pharmaceutical industries. Causes digestive conditions, damage to the human immune system, skin irritations, swelling and sensitivity to joints. Also causes respiratory problems and asphyxia. Can lead to cancer. Is linked to: '*endocrine disruption, neurotoxicity*[202] *weakens the immune system.*'[203] Approved in the United States, European Union, New Zealand and Australia**. Avoid**

| 575 <br> **Safe** or **Caution** <br> | **Glucono delta-lactone(GDL) or Gluconolactone** |
|---|---|

**Colour: White odourless crystalline powder**
Used in commercially made food products. Used as an acidifier, artificial sweetener, leavening agent, food acid

---

[202] Brain and neuron damage.
[203] http://thearticlebay.com

and acidity regulator, also used as a sequestrant.[204] Can be derived from genetically modified maize. Is made from glucose.[205] Can be used for curing and pickling. Can be a naturally occurring food product found in many foods. GDL is added to feta cheese, honey, fruit juices, wine, processed meat and gluten-free food products. Can also be found in fish, prawns, grape juice, bean products, sausages and in fish and meat paste. Can damage the intestinal lining. Approved in the United States, European Union, New Zealand and Australia. Safe or Caution

| 576 Avoid | Sodium gluconate |
|---|---|

**Colour: White to tan fine or granular crystalline powder**
Is a gluconic acid of 574. Used as a sequestrant, stabiliser and thickener. Is a synthetic additive added to many food products. Picks up metal traces, binds them in the product to form a shellation.[206] Products include: dietary and nutritional supplements, baked goods, soft confectionary, sweets and lollies, fizzy/carbonated drinks, desserts and processed meats. Is also added to baby and infant formulas, snacks and cereals, flavour enhancers, fruit and vegetables, ready-made meals, fast food, salad dressing, seasoning, sauces, relishes and tabletop products, tea, coffee and added to water treatment. Reactions can include: chest pains, feeling of passing out, flushing, uneven heart rate, high blood pressure, severe headaches, blurred vision, buzzing in the ears and anxiety attacks. Can lead to intestinal damage. Approved in the United States, European Union and New Zealand. Banned in Australia. Avoid

---

[204] A food additive that improves the quality of the food.
[205] A simple sugar which is a component of many carbohydrates.
[206] A particular way that ions and molecules bind metal ions.

| 577 **Caution** or **Avoid** | Potassium gluconate |
|---|---|

**Colour: White crystalline powder**
A synthetic mineral supplement and sequestrant. Is used as a food additive, acidity regulator and yeast in manufactured food products. Is also the potassium salt of gluconic acid. Is used in many dietary supplements. Can damage the intestinal lining, lead to stomach pain, gas, diarrhoea, vomiting, confusion and anxiety, uneven heart beat, muscle weakness, cramping, numbness in the hands or feet and nausea. Picks up metal traces, binds them in the product to form a shellation. May be used for treating low levels of calcium. Approved in the United States, the European Union, New Zealand. Banned in Australia. **Caution** or **Avoid**

| 578 **Caution** or **Avoid** | Calcium gluconate |
|---|---|

**Colour: White free-flowing salt**
Is a synthesised additive used as a sequestrant, firming and buffer agent in a large range of food products, including: meat, cheese, pudding powders, custards, canned vegetables, bakery products and infant milk formulas. Is also used as an artificial sweetener. Can cause damage to the intestinal lining, heart problems and is linked to 'brain disorders.'[207] See 574 gluconic acid, The Article Bay. May pick up metal traces and bind them in the product. May not be compatible with other medications. Approved in the United States, European Union, New Zealand and Australia. **Caution** or **Avoid**

---

[207] http://thearticlebay.com

| 579 Avoid | Ferrous gluconate |
|---|---|

**Colour: Fine yellow to green powder**
A form of mineral iron combined with glucose. Is a food colouring agent and food stabiliser used in iron supplements, mineral tablets and vitamins. Is used to maintain the pigment in olives. May be safe in small quantities. Is used in fortified food and in baby food. May be labelled as iron in manufactured foods including baby formula. Can cause stomach discomfort, gastrointestinal problems, lung irritation and the inability to regulate iron absorption. Excessive exposure to iron can bring on the onset of hemochromatosis – enlarged body organs, which can lead to ill health and death. Exposure for children under twenty four months, can cause death. Restricted only in the use of olives in the United States. Approved in the United States, European Union, New Zealand and Australia. **Avoid**

| 580 Caution or Avoid | Magnesium glucomate |
|---|---|

**Colour: Off-white to white powder**
A magnesium salt of gluconic acid and produced by the fermentation of carbohydrates. The commercial additive may be synthetic, check the labelling. Is used as a food flavour enhancer, acidity regulator and firming agent. Natural gluconate is often found in naturally fermented wine, fruit and honey. More research is needed into the food value of this additive. On alert in the United States. Not permitted in the European Union. Approved in New Zealand and Australia. **Caution** or **Avoid**

| 586 Avoid | 4-Hexylresorcinol |
|-----------|-------------------|

**Colour: White organic powder**

'*Is produced by sulphonating benzene with fuming sulphuric acid and fusing the resulting benzenedisulfonic acid with caustic soda.*'[208] Is an organic compound with local anaesthetic, antiseptic and anthelmintic[209] properties. Used as an antioxidant in throat lozenges and in the extension of shelf life for shrimp and possibly other saleable sea food. Is linked to '*endocrine disruption, cancer and toxic to the reproductive system.*'[210] Linked to a range of health problems including reduced sperm count in males and the risk of breast cancer in women. See additive 310, page 215. On alert in the United States. Approved in the European Union, New Zealand and Australia. **Avoid**

---

[208] http://www.wotzinurfood.com
[209] Used to destroy parasitic worms.
[210] http://thearticlebay.com

**Your Notes**

**Devils:** Flavour enhancers, glutamates and glutamate boosters **(600 range)**

Frequently hidden as yeast extract, hydrolysed vegetable protein (HVP) or hydrolysed plant protein (HPP)

| Devil Numbers | Additive |
|---|---|
| **620**<br>**Avoid** | **L-glutamic acid** |

**Colour: Colourless or white crystalline powder**
Is commercially prepared by bacterial fermentation from molasses. Is a synthetic additive. Can be manufactured from gluten vegetable protein or soy protein. Commercially derived from unbound amino acids.[211] Is used as a bulking agent in bread and bakery goods and as a flavour enhancer. Is a salt substitute, glazing agent, foaming agent and humectant. Used in sausages, seasoning, savoury snacks, sardines, tomatoes, Chinese and other Asian foods. Will increase appetite and contribute to eating disorders and obesity. Will also contribute to: '*ADD (attention deficit disorder) ADHD (attention deficit hyperactivity disorder), brain damage (destroys brain cells in the hypothalamus), convulsions, depression, personality disorders, paranoia, schizophrenia, learning and memory difficulties, uncontrolled anger, liver damage, headaches.'*[212] Could kill nerve cells resulting in the onset

---

[211] Found naturally in various foods, L-glutamic acid is a naturally occurring amino acid. Additive 620 is a manufactured unbound chemical containing L-glutamic acid and dangerous pollutants. Such pollutants contain D-glutamic acid, a proven neuropoison, pyroglutamin acid and other harmful pullutants such as mono-and dichlopropnols which are not removable from the human system. Ref: The Article Bay.
[212] http://thearticlebay.com

of Huntington's and Parkinson's disease. Babies and children should avoid. Similar effects to MSG. A dangerous synthetic additive that should be banned. Approved in the United States, European Union, New Zealand and Australia. **Avoid**

| 621<br>**Avoid** | **Monosodium L-glutamate or MSG** |
|---|---|

**Colour: Odourless, Crystalline Powder**
Is a sodium salt from 620. A synthetic derived from molasses by bacterial fermentation. Is used in bread and bakery goods as a flavour enhancer. Used as a low-sodium salt substitute in many commercially produced food products. Is also added to any 'dead, poor or bad tasting' processed foods. Used in canned tuna, canned vegetables, sausages, cracker biscuits, instant noodles, soups, stock cubes, dressings, potato chips, pre-packed meals, snacks and Chinese and Asian meals. Will cause headaches, dizziness, nausea, neck pain, migraine, asthma, hyperactivity and behavioural problems including ADD, ADHD and other behavioural changes. Can be a factor in insomnia and increase appetite contributing to obesity problems. Is linked to neurological disorders including Alzheimer's, Huntington's and Parkinson's diseases. Not suitable for babies, young children, pregnant or lactating women. A dangerous synthetic additive that should be banned. See 620. Approved in the United States, European Union, New Zealand and Australia. **Avoid**

| 622<br>Avoid | Monopotassium L-glutamate |
|---|---|

**Colour: White crystalline powder**

Is a synthetic and commercially prepared additive by bacterial fermentation of molasses. Is used as a bulking agent in bread and bakery goods, also used as a flavour enhancer. Also prepared from vegetable protein such as soy or gluten. Glutamates can have a umami[213] taste and enhance many different flavours thus reducing the quantity of salt required. Added to a great number of processed foods, including: canned vegetables, canned tuna, frozen foods, dressings, potato chips, crisps and stock cubes. Is used in over 10,000 processed foods in the United States. Used in weight loss foods and drinks which will often give the reverse effect – people gain weight because of the effects of the additive! Will cause hypersensitive reactions in some people. Can lead to behavioural problems, depression, gastrointestinal conditions, headaches, migraine and contribute to learning difficulties. Has been linked to Huntington's, Alzheimer's and Parkinson's diseases. Will also cause urticaria, insomnia, abdominal cramps, nausea, vomiting, diarrhoea, allergic reactions, including asthma. Harmful to people with kidney stones or kidney conditions, heart conditions and pregnant women. Should not be given to infants and small children as it may contribute to damage of the nervous system. A dangerous synthetic additive that should be avoided or banned. See 620. Approved in the United States, European Union, New Zealand and Australia. **Avoid**

---

[213] A distinctive and pleasant, savoury taste experienced through taste receptors. Experiences usually relate to broths, cooked meats or those foods containing monosodium glutamates (MSG).

| 623 Avoid | Calcium di-L-glutamate |
|---|---|

**Colour: White odourless crystals**

A synthetic bulking agent, flavour and bread enhancer and humectant. Used as a salt substitute. Possibly a genetically modified product prepared from molasses by bacterial fermentation. This becomes the calcium salt from glutamic acid. Also used in animal food, cigarettes and up to 10,000 commercially prepared foods in the United States. Also used in canned vegetables and tuna, stock cubes, salad dressings, potato crisps and chips and a wide range of frozen foods. There may be adverse reactions in asthmatics. Contributes to allergic and hypersensitive reactions, behavioural problems, learning difficulties, depression, gastrointestinal ailments, headaches and migraine. Not permitted in foods for babies and young children as it has the potential to damage the nervous system. May be linked to Parkinson's, Huntington's and Alzheimer's diseases. *'Pregnant women, children, hypoglycaemic, elderly and those with heart disease are at risk from reactions. Dangerous chemical additive.'*[214] Should be banned. See 620. On alert in the United States. Approved in the European Union, New Zealand and Australia. **Avoid**

| 624 Avoid | Monoammonium L-glutamate |
|---|---|

**Colour: Colourless, odourless crystal**

From molasses and through bacterial fermentation is a synthetic, commercially derived, food additive, enhancer and salt substitute. See 620. Is used as a bulking agent in

---

[214] http://www.wotzinurfood.com

bread and bakery goods, also used as a flavour enhancer. Commercially prepared from soy and gluten. Used in gravies, glazing agents, brewer's yeast, rice protein, corn starch, chewing gum, added to some milk as a protein. Also added to long-life milk, milk powder, milk shakes and malt flavouring, yeast extract spreads, cheese yogurts, gelatine, some vegetarian food, meat, chicken, oysters, pork, shrimp and seafood for flavouring. Is added to potato starch, protein bars, soy extract foods, seasoning and vegetarian rennet. Read the labels of the foods before you buy. May contribute to asthma, depression, gastrointestinal complaints, headaches, migraine and learning difficulties. May also contribute to ADHD and behavioural problems. Pregnant women, children, people suffering from heart conditions should avoid. Is a dangerous additive and should be banned. Approved in the United States, European Union, New Zealand and Australia. **Avoid**

| 625<br>**Avoid**<br> | **Magnesium glutamate** |
| --- | --- |

**Colour: White or off-white crystalline powder**
Is a synthetic additive derived from the fermentation of molasses. Is a magnesium acid salt of glutamic acid. Used as a bulking, enhancement and humectant in bread and bakery products. As a salt substitute, is used as a flavour enhancer that is found in many commercially prepared savoury foods including: frozen foods, canned tuna, canned vegetable, stock cubes, crisps, chips and potato-based snacks. May contribute to: *'ADD (attention deficit disorder) ADHD (attention deficit hyperactivity disorder), eating and obesity disorders, brain damage (destroys brain cells in the hypothalamus), convulsions, depression, personality disorders, paranoia, schizophrenia, learning and memory difficulties, uncontrolled anger, liver damage, headaches, birth defects, female hormonal disorders, high*

*blood sugars, and anxiety.*[215] Also linked to: Alzheimer's, Huntington's and Parkinson's diseases. May also be linked to other, as yet, undiscovered illnesses or conditions. See 620. Should be avoided or permanently banned. On alert in the United States. Approved in the European Union, New Zealand and Australia. **Avoid**

| 627 **Avoid** | Disodium-5'-guanylate also known as: Sodium 5'-guanylate and disodium 5' guanylate |
|---|---|

**Colour: White crystalline or crystal powder**
Used as a flavour enhancer, bulking agent and bread enhancer. Is extracted from yeast, seaweed, pigs or fish and possibly sardines. Can be produced from genetically modified life forms or organisms. Used in instant noodles, corn chips, rice crackers, Chinese foods, soups, sausage rolls, some instant mashed potatoes, stuffing in some frozen chickens and turkeys, gravies, salad dressings, salsa flavouring in tuna, stocks and stock cubes, pasta meals including macaroni cheese, marinated meats from the local butcher, commercially produced sausages, fast foods including: chicken and chips, some fresh chickens and sea food extenders. May cause behavioural problems, skin irritation, asthma, gastrointestinal irritability, headaches, itching, dizziness, chest pain, gout in some people and hives. Not safe for babies and young children. Can be a dangerous additive for those people who suffer with any form of kidney or related conditions or people sensitive to purines.[216] Approved in the United States, European Union, New Zealand and Australia. **Avoid**

---

[215] http://thearticlebay.com
[216] A crystalline, colourless compound, on oxidation forms uric acid.

| 631 Avoid | Disodium-5'-inosinate |
|---|---|

**Colour: White crystal or crystalline powder**

A synthetic additive commercially produced from a microbial base of vegetable sources. Also produced from meat or fish (sardines). Is used as a bulking agent, flavour and bread enhancer and glazing agent. May also be produced by the bacterial fermentation of sugars. Used in instant noodles, potato chips, savoury snacks and biscuits, savoury rice, tinned vegetables, cured meats and packet soups. Allergic and hypersensitive reaction may occur including behavioural problems, gastrointestinal ailments, headaches, migraine, irritation to the skin, eczema, dermatitis, itching, hives, rashes and sleep disturbance. May trigger gout symptoms. Can be dangerous for people who suffer from kidney problems or those that react to purines. Not permitted in foods for infants and young children. Not recommended for pregnant or lactating mothers. Can be a commercially exploited additive. If possible, check label for origin of ingredients. Approved in the United States, European Union, New Zealand and Australia. **Avoid**

| 635 Avoid | Disodium-5'-ribonucleotides |
|---|---|

**Colour: White crystalline powder**

A food enhancer also known as an inosinate[217] – a synthetic, possibly made from genetically modified ingredients, used as a flavour enhancer in the food and beverage industry. May be extracted from yeast or fish. In

---

[217] A food enhancer that enhances flavour. Flavourless (dead food) can be made to look and taste delicious by many additives.

the United States nucleotide[218] is extracted from torula[219] yeast which is grown on alcohol. Nucleotide is used in the production of infant formula. This additive is also used in Chinese food, instant noodles, corn chips, flavoured barbeque chicken, biscuits, rice crackers, packet and canned soups, party pies, sausage rolls, some instant mashed potatoes, stuffing in some frozen chickens and turkeys, gravies, salad dressings, salsa flavouring in tuna, stocks and stock cubes, pasta meals including macaroni cheese, marinated meats from the local butcher, commercially produced sausages, fast foods and take away foods, including: chicken and chips, some fresh chickens and *sea food extenders*[220]. Will cause behavioural problems, skin irritation, asthma, gastrointestinal irritability, headaches, itching, dizziness, chest pain and hives. *'Dangerous for children and young people and those suffering from kidney disorders and all medical conditions that require the avoidance of purines.'*[221] Additive 620-625, are almost never listed on the food ingredients panel of the product. Is banned in some countries. See 626. Please note[222] on alert in the United States. Approved in the European Union, New Zealand and Australia. **Avoid**

---

[218] A compound linked to a phosphate group.

[219] A yeast which is cultured and grown for use as an additive or for medicines.

[220] https://www.fedup.com.au

[221] http://thearticlebay.com

[222] 635 is a combination of 627 and 631. Is a yeast extract, hydrolysed vegetable protein (HVP) and hydrolysed plant protein (HPP) are ways the food manufacturer can include MSG without having to declare it on the food label.

| 636 **Avoid** | Maltol |
|---|---|

**Colour: White crystalline powder**
Originally, an organic compound found in the bark of larch trees, pine needles and roasted malt. Can be synthetically produced. Is not registered as a food additive. Is used as a flavour enhancer and enhances the aroma of freshly baked bread. Gives a fresh baked taste to bread and cakes. Enhances the flavour of chocolate substitutes, soft and fizzy drinks, ice cream, confectionary, jams and conserves. Can increase the body's ability to absorb aluminium. *'It can help aluminium pass to the brain causing Alzheimer's disease.'* [223] May contribute to cardiovascular disorders and ill health. May also lead to hyperactivity, urticaria, asthma and insomnia. On alert in the United States and the European Union. Approved in New Zealand and Australia.
**Avoid**

| 637 | Ethyl maltol |
|---|---|

**Colour: White crystalline powder**
Is a synthetic chemically derived from maltol. Is used as a bulking and glazing agent. Also used to produce the aroma of bread and bakery goods. Used in gluten-free food to enhance the flavour. Has the ability to extend the shelf life date of many foods. Is widely used in the food and beverage industries. Is used in pasta, sauces, baked goods, including bakery products. 637 thickens and binds products together. Not safe for babies or infants. May cause urticaria and insomnia. Pregnant and lactating mothers should avoid. More research is required on this

---

[223] https://noshly.com

additive. On alert in the United States and European Union. Approved in New Zealand and Australia. **Avoid**

| 640 **Caution** or **Avoid** | Glycine |
|---|---|

**Colour: Crystalline solid**
Is mainly derived from gelatine, (possibly from animal bones) and is partially synthetic. Origin of the product needs to be identified. Is a genetically coded amino acid. Is used as a food enhancer, bulking and glazing agent. Is mainly used in bread, bakery and dietary products. Is mildly toxic. See 620. Approved in the United States, European Union, New Zealand and Australia. **Caution** or **Avoid**

| 641 **Avoid** | L-Leucine |
|---|---|

**Colour: White crystalline powder**
Is a flavour enhancer and food modifier. Is a natural amino acid and building block of protein. In commercial production is synthetic manufactured using a chemical process. Mainly produced from gelatine which may be derived from animal bones. Used in bread, bakery products and health foods including dietary supplements. Can result in kidney and liver damage. Not advisable during pregnancy or for lactating mothers. Do not give to babies and young children. Laboratory testing caused birth defects in animals. Can be very toxic if ingested. Approved in the United States. On alert in the European Union. Approved in New Zealand and Australia. **Avoid**

**Your Notes**

...........................................................................

...........................................................................

...........................................................................

...........................................................................

...........................................................................

...........................................................................

...........................................................................

...........................................................................

...........................................................................

...........................................................................

...........................................................................

...........................................................................

...........................................................................

...........................................................................

...........................................................................

...........................................................................

...........................................................................

...........................................................................

...........................................................................

...........................................................................

# Devils: Miscellaneous additives (900 range)

| Devil Numbers | Additive |
|---|---|

| 900a<br>Avoid | Polydimethylsiloxane or Dimethylpolysiloxane (PDMS) |
|---|---|

**Colour: Light viscous liquid**

Is a miscellaneous flavour enhancer. Is silicone-based, water repellent, anti-foaming agent used as an emulsifier, anti-caking agent which is added to many cooking oils that are widely used in the global, fast-food industry. Prevents the oil from foaming allowing it to last longer, this reduces costs while the food is cooked in old oil. May be combined with additive 319 to keep food shape. Can contain formaldehyde.[224] Is used in the manufacture of: French fries, hash browns, milk shakes, smoothies, confectionary, chocolate, syrups, soft drinks, cordials, toppings, instant coffee, vinegar and chewing gum. Is linked to cancer. 900a has not been fully evaluated. Approved in the United States, European Union, New Zealand and Australia. **Avoid**

| 901<br>Safe or Caution | Beeswax |
|---|---|

**Colour: Whit to yellow**

Is a natural product produced by bees within their hives. Is used as a glazing agent to wax fruit. Also used in many areas of confectionary including: ice cream, chocolate and snack food. Also used in slow-release pills. Will occasionally

---

[224] Made from oxidizing the vapour of methanol. Widely used in the wood industry. Is declared a carcinogen by the International Agency for Research on Cancer.

cause an allergic reaction. Approved in the United States, European Union, New Zealand and Australia. Safe or Caution

| 903 Caution or Avoid | Carnauba wax |
|---|---|

**Colour: Hard yellow brown flakes**
Known as the Queen of wax comes from the leaves of the palm, Copernicia prunifera. Is used as a glazing agent to wax fruit, to produce the shine in chocolate production and to give the shine in confectionary coatings. Is used to coat sweets, candies, mint sweets, frosting and in some sauces. Used in cocoa products. Also used as a flavour carrier in drinks, savoury snacks and toppings. Used in tablet coating for the pharmaceutical industry. When combined with coconut oil is also used in shoe wax, polishes, paper and surfboard coatings. Can cause allergies in sensitive people. Can cause eczema and is a possible carcinogen. Approved in the United States, European Union, New Zealand and Australia. Caution or Avoid

| 904 Caution or Avoid | Shellac |
|---|---|

**Colour: Off-white to tan granular resin**
Shellac is a sticky resin excretion from the Kerria lacca beetle. The beetle uses the excretion to stick to trees. In commercial use, once harvested, the resin is bleached to off-white to tan. May be mixed with ethanol when used in glazing of confectionary. Check your supplier's information. Is used as a glazing agent in the food industry. Is used in confectionery, including: lollies, high

gloss, (jelly-type) surface-based jelly beans, chocolate beans and drops and a variety of different chocolate confectionary. Eaten by millions of people around the world. Also used in orange fizzy drinks and orange skin medications. Shellac is a hardy natural primer, sanding agent used in wooden furniture making. May cause allergic skin reactions and eczema. On alert in the United States, approved in the European Union, New Zealand and Australia. **Caution** or **Avoid**

| 905<br>**Avoid** | **Petroleum wax c<br>(i) Microcrystalline wax<br>(ii) Paraffin wax** |
|---|---|

**Colour: White mineral oil produced from hydrocarbons**

A by-product and synthetic additive produced from petroleum. Also known as mineral oil, petroleum jelly, paraffin, paraffin wax and paraffin oil. Also used in health care products. Is used as an ingredient in chewing gum and as a protective coating on fruit and vegetables. Used in sweets, lollies or candies, a wide range of confectionary, in and on dried fruit. Also used in yeast production and as a binder and coating for tablets and capsules. May be linked to bowel cancer and intestinal disorders. May inhibit natural food vitamins, the absorption of fat soluble vitamins and other food benefits. May have teratogenic properties.[225] May work as a laxative. Can have severe allergic reactions. Is used in teeth floss. Approved in the United States (ii). On alert in the United States petroleum wax c and (i). All are on alert in the European Union, New Zealand and Australia. **Avoid**

---

[225] A factor or cause which brings about the malformation of an embryo.

| 905b **Avoid** | Petroleum or Petroleum jelly |
|---|---|

**Colour: Light yellow jelly**
Petroleum jelly is a synthesized product made from hydrocarbons extracted from petroleum products. Is used as a protective coating on fresh fruit and vegetables to make them look shiny and appealing whilst protecting them from spoilage. Also used as a glazing on chocolate, sweets and confectionary. Causes allergic skin reactions. When eaten, can inhibit absorption of natural digestive fats. Has been linked to cancer. Approved in the United States. On alert in the European Union. Approved in New Zealand and Australia. **Avoid**

| 914 **Avoid** | Oxidised polyethylene |
|---|---|

**Colour: Waxing agent**
Is an ethylene polymer produced from petroleum. Is used as an humectant and glazing agent in the food industry. Oxidised polyethylene wax is '*authorised for the surface treatment of some fruits.*'[226] Is linked to cancer. Check for approval in the United States and New Zealand. Approved in the European Union and Australia. **Avoid**

---

[226] https://www.efsa.europa.eu

| 920<br>**Avoid** | L-cysteine<br>monohydrochloride |
|---|---|

**Colour: White Crystalline powder**
Is a synthesized and unbound chemical which is manufactured for use in the food industry. Is produced from bird feathers, animal hair, including hog hair, if from China, and human hair. Is widely used as a food supplement. Is used as a food enhancer. Also used in flour as it stabilises the structure of leavened bread. Used in chicken flavouring. Aids in detoxification of chemicals, including smoking, prevents brain and liver damage due to too much alcohol consumption. Is also linked to *'endocrine disruption, cancer, disorders of the reproductive system, brain and nervous system damage.'*[227] Is a known neurotoxin. Seek medical help before consumption of this product. Approved in the United States, European Union, New Zealand and Australia. **Avoid**

| 925<br>**Avoid** | Chlorine |
|---|---|

**Colour: Clear, yellow liquid**
The vapour releases a green to yellow gas. Is used as a preservative. Destroys natural nutrients. Used in municipal tap water and as a compound bleaching agent in flour. Is used as a disinfectant, deodoriser and decolouriser. Is a known carcinogen. Can cause serious lung damage if inhaled. May cause burning to the skin. Is on alert in the United States, European Union, New Zealand and Australia. **Avoid**

---

[227] http://thearticlebay.com

| 926 **Avoid** | Chlorine dioxide |
|---|---|

**Colour: Solid, colourless and odourless**
An additive derived from urea (urine) producing ammonia. (a) and (b) which are used as improving agents in a number of products. Is used as a compounding agent to treat flour, also used as a browning agent in bakery bread and dough products. 927b is used as a nutrient in fermented products. Contains formaldehyde. Is linked to *cancer, genetic damage and birth defects.*[228] Approved in the United States and the European Union. On alert in New Zealand and Australia. **Avoid**

| 928 **Caution** or **Avoid** | Benzole peroxide |
|---|---|

**Colour: Colourless and crystalline solid**
Is used in the bleaching of caroteniods in white, refined bread flour. Also used for bleaching teeth and hair. Used in the production of polymerising polyester; has many other commercial uses. See 210. Will affect asthmatic sufferers and those people with allergies. Approved in the United States. On alert in the European Union, New Zealand and Australia. **Caution** or **Avoid**

---

[228] http://thearticlebay.com

## Your Notes

# Devils: Propellants (900 range)

| Devil Numbers | Additive |
|---|---|
| **941** <br> Safe | **Nitrogen** |

**Colour: Colourless, odourless, tasteless, non-toxic and chemically inert gas**

Is used to displace moisture and oxygen in packaging. It also extends the shelf life of perishable goods. Nitrogen is used in Modified Atmosphere Packaging, (MAP). It expels food from a container as in whipped cream. Is also used in beer to create smallish bubbles and smoothness. Is used in vacuum packaging to reduce spoilage, yeast and bacterial attack. Also used to transport perishable products from distant countries. Used in: corn chips, snacks, nuts, fresh and chilled meats, poultry and fish, cooked meats, palm and coconut oils, potato chips, powdered milk, spices, dried products including fruit, Pita bread, Naan bread, pizza bases, grated cheese, dairy products, fruit juices, wine, salads and fresh vegetables. Considered safe at this point. Buying locally produced food will eliminate the use of nitrogen in packaging. Excessive release of nitrogen in a confined environment can prove fatal. Approved in the United States, European Union, New Zealand and Australia. Safe

| Devil Numbers | Additive |
|---|---|
| **942** <br> Avoid | **Nitrous oxide** |

**Colour: Colourless, odourless gas**

Also known as laughing gas, mainly used in the medical industry. In the food industry, it protects food from deterioration and oxidation. Is also used as a foaming

343

agent to solidify food. Is used in the canisters for whipped cream, cooking oils and sprays. Will inhibit growth in cut, packaged potatoes, potato chips and similar food prepared for the supermarket shelves. Used as a packaging gas for distance delivery. Is linked to *'cancer and birth defects'*.[229] In confined spaces and from nitrous oxide, a person may experience the following: headache, dizziness, drowsiness, vomiting and ringing in the ears. Is highly toxic. Approved in the United States, European Union, New Zealand and Australia. **Avoid**

| 943a<br>**Avoid** | Butane |
|---|---|

**Colour: Flammable, colourless, easily liquefied gas.**
A highly propellant liquid gas in aerosol cans containing vegetable-based and water-based emulsion cooking oils for baking and frying, mocked cream and food velveting effects for frozen desserts. Is a petroleum derivative. Has caused cancer in laboratory testing on animals. Can contribute to severe allergic reactions. Approved in the United States, European Union, New Zealand and Australia. **Avoid**

| 943b<br>**Avoid** | Isobutane |
|---|---|

**Colour: Also known as methylpropane**
Is a neurotoxic, at high concentration on the NIH[230] hazards list. Is a gas propellant which expels food from a

---

[229] http://thearticlebay.com
[230] National Institutes of Health.

container; found in spray cans. May bring on severe allergic reactions. May induce headaches, dizziness, ringing in the ears, drowsiness, nausea and vomiting. Approved in the United States, European Union, New Zealand and Australia. **Avoid**

| 944 **Avoid** | Propane |
|---|---|

**Colour: Natural inert gas**
Used as a propellant in the food industry. Is a by-product of petroleum refining and a toxic substance. Used in aerosol sprays and deodorants. Approved in the United States, European Union, New Zealand and Australia. **Avoid**

| 946 **Caution** or **Avoid** | Octafluorocyclobutane or Perfluorocyclobutane |
|---|---|

**Colour: A colourless non-flammable gas**
Is a member of the food packaging and propellant group. Is an aerating agent in foam or sprayed food products. Propels food from the container. Has derived from hydride of cyclobutane.[231] More research is needed to long-term health effects and outcomes. Approved in the United States. On alert in the European Union. Approved in Australia. **Caution** or **Avoid**

---

[231] A binary compound of hydrogen with a metal

**Your Notes**

.......................................................................................

.......................................................................................

.......................................................................................

.......................................................................................

.......................................................................................

.......................................................................................

.......................................................................................

.......................................................................................

.......................................................................................

.......................................................................................

.......................................................................................

.......................................................................................

.......................................................................................

.......................................................................................

.......................................................................................

.......................................................................................

.......................................................................................

.......................................................................................

.......................................................................................

.......................................................................................

**Devils: Artificial sweeteners (900 range)**

The health benefits or safety of these products has not been adequately proven. In some instances, additives labelled as 'diet', 'light', 'lite' or with a similar name have been found to increase weight gain and not reduce it.

| Devil Numbers | Additive |
|---|---|
| **950**<br>**Avoid** | **Acesulphame potassium** |

**Colour: White crystalline powder**
Is a high-intensity, non-caloric, synthetic sweetener. Is at least 200 times sweeter than sucrose (sugar). It has many different names: Acesulfame potassium, Ace-K, Sunette and Sweet One. Is used in frozen desserts, sweets, candies, confectionary, lollies, chewing gum, instant powdered drinks, low-joule gums, in many diet foods and commercially produced baked products. Is used across a range of dairy products. Laboratory testing has shown tumours of the lung, mammary glands, rare formations of the thymus, leukaemia and cancer in test animals. *'The Center for Science in the Public Interest (CSPI) includes the artificial sweeteners: aspartame, saccharine and acesulfame* (Acesulphame) *K as part of the Ten Worst Additives.'*[232] Please note: many synthetic sweeteners have the additive 950. Is linked to cancer in humans. Approved in the United States, European Union, New Zealand and Australia. **Avoid**
Further notes[233]

---

[232] http://www.healthynutritionguide.info

[233] In chemical structure, acesulfame potassium is the potassium salt of 6-methyl-1,2,3-oxathiazine-4(3H)-one 2,2-dioxide.

| 951<br>Avoid | Aspartame<br>Nutrasweet<br>Equal |
|---|---|

**Colour: White granule or powder**

Is a synthetic, non-saccharide, flavour enhancer and sweetener. May be manufactured from genetically modified micro-organisms (Escherichia coli). Used in bread, spreads, carbonated soft drinks, frozen desserts, toppings, fillings, puddings, jellies, breakfast cereals, jams, marmalades, sweets, lollies, confectionary, hot chocolate powder, multivitamins, powdered soft drinks, chewing gum and some pharmaceutical medications. '*Aspartame is linked to many health problems including: 'dizziness, insomnia, vision problems, slurred speech, apoplexy,[234] causes in brain chemistry and behaviour, neurological disorders, menstrual problems, brain tumours and seizures, brain damage, birth defects, epileptic seizures, deep depression, cancer and severe headaches.'*[235] Not safe for asthmatics, may cause allergies. (The Food and Drug Administration (FDA), USA. have recorded 92 different symptoms related to Aspartame.) It has been used in low-cal or sugar-free foods since 1974. A dangerous chemical that should be banned. Many synthetic sweeteners contain 951. Approved in the United States, European Union, New Zealand and Australia. **Avoid**

---

[234] An incapacity to remain conscious resulting from a cerebral haemorrhage or stroke.
[235] http://thearticlebay.com

| 952 Avoid | Cyclamates:<br>(i) Cyclamatic acid<br>(ii) Calcium cyclamate<br>(iii) Potassium cyclamate<br>(iv) Sodium cyclamate |
| --- | --- |

**Colour: White colourless crystals or crystalline powder**

Is the calcium salt of cyclamic acid which incorporates a reaction with sulfamic acid[236] and cyclohexylamine.[237] A consequence with cyclohexylamine with either sulfamic acid or sulphur trioxide creates the artificial sweetener of sodium cyclamate. Used in many soft, fizzy, fruit and diet drinks. Used in tabletop sweeteners, some baking and other manufactured and cooked foods. Known to cause headaches and some migraines. Can be a carcinogen. Has been linked to bladder and liver damage, birth defects, testicular cancer and sterility. Also known to cause testicular damage to rats in animal studies and research. Still available in the United Kingdom. Banned in the United States and European Union. Approved for use in New Zealand and Australia. **Avoid**

| 953 Caution or Avoid | Isomalt |
| --- | --- |

**Colour: An odourless, white crystalline substance**

Is a synthetic sweetener prepared from a combination of sugar alcohols: gluco mannitol and gluco sorbitol derived from genetically modified sugar beet. The process includes

---

[236] A strong crystalline acid compound used in weed killer and cleaning agents.

[237] An organic base, with a corrosion inhibitor, used in the production of rubber and plastics.

the hydrogenation[238] between the beet molecules; through the catalyst of heating metal rods of either: nickel, palladium or platinum. The process hydrogenation is not compatible with the human digestive and gut system. Through evolution, we have not developed the gut enzymes to cope with hydrogenated food products. Is used in sugar-free sweets, candy, toffees, lollipops, fudge, cough lollies and drops, wafers, throat lozenges, lollies and in sugar sculpture for decoration in cakes and confectionary. Not permitted in infant food. Is linked to diarrhoea, gas and stomach discomfort. On alert in the United States. Approved in the European Union and New Zealand. Not listed for use in Australia. **Caution** or **Avoid**

| 954<br>**Avoid** | Saccharins or<br>**(i) Saccharin**<br>**(ii) Calcium Saccharin**<br>**(iii) Potassium saccharin**<br>**(iv) Sodium saccharin** |
|---|---|

**Colour: White powder of sodium salt**
A synthetic, artificial sweetener. Originally derived from toluene (a known carcinogen) a product of pine oil discovered in 1837 by Flip Walter. Further research lead to the discovery of a hydrocarbon which is related to the benzene family. Is also extracted from coal tar. Used to sweeten drinks, sweets, candies, confectionary, biscuits, medicines and toothpaste. Toluene interferes with normal blood coagulation, blood sugar levels and the digestive function. Is linked to many conditions including: testicular cancer, birth defects, cancer and genetic damage. Banned in France, Germany, Hungary, Portugal and Spain. Also banned as a food additive in Malaysia and Zimbabwe and banned as a beverage additive in Fiji, Israel, Peru and Taiwan. Approved in the United States. Not approved in

---

[238] Hydrogenation reduces the natural structure of the molecule to a hydrocarbon.

the European Union (ii) calcium saccharin. All approved in New Zealand and Australia. **Avoid**

| 955<br>**Avoid** | Sucralose<br>**(Trichlorogalactosucrose)** |
|---|---|

**Colour: White crystalline powder**
Is manufactured by chlorinating sugar/sucrose. Sucralose can contain small particles of heavy metals, methanol and arsenic. May be processed through hydrogenation. Laboratory testing has shown neurological and immunological disorders. Caused kidney and liver damage and detrimental effects to the thalamus glands and renal mineralisation. Has also been linked to: *'depression, diarrhoea, dizziness, enlarged kidneys, gas, headaches, irregular heartbeat, migraines, miscarriages, muscle pain, nausea, panic disorder, pre-menstrual tension (PMS), reduced growth, reduction in the number of blood cells, reduced thymus gland, stomach pain and weight gain.'*[239] From the information given, this additive may stimulate the 'pleasure centre' of the brain, please see page 23. Is suspected to be neurotoxic and be anti-fertility. The Centre for Science in the Public Interest, (CSPI) has downgraded this additive from **Safe** to **Avoid**. Also see[240] Approved in the United States, European Union, New Zealand and Australia. **Avoid**

---

[239] http://thearticlebay.com
[240] For further information about the product: www.truthaboutsplenda.com

| 956 **Avoid** | Alitame |
|---|---|

**Colour: White crystalline powder**
Artificial sweetener at least 2,000 times sweeter than sugar. Is used in a wide range of food including: chewing gum, beverages, in a wide distribution of bakery products, water-based flavoured drinks, dairy-based drinks, cream and ice cream, jams, and a range of confectionary. Causes aggravated liver abnormalities in laboratory testing. *Recent research reveals sweeteners do not help with weight control*. New research suggests that, '*...sweeteners affect the bacteria in the bowel in adverse ways thus impairing glucose metabolism.*'[241] On alert in the United States and in the European Union. Approved in New Zealand and Australia. **Avoid**

| 957 **Avoid** | Thaumatin |
|---|---|

**Colour: Light-gold liquid**
Is also known as talin. Is extracted from the arils[242] of the Katemfe fruit (Thaumatococcus daniellii Bennett). Is composed of two proteins, some of which are 2,000 times sweeter than sucrose (table sugar). Is related to the dangerous additive 620[243] which can include pathogens. Is used as a food and flavour enhancer. Also used to sweeten wines, included in some vitamin tablets, commercially baked foods, dairy products, breads of many types, fruit

---

[241] https://www.sciencenews.org
[242] Extra seed covering – can be fleshy or hairy.
[243] http://thearticlebay.com

and chewing gum. Also used in confectionary products, diet drinks, gummy lollies or sweets, juices, coffee and yogurts. May be responsible for a number of health problems including: ADHD, ADD, nerve cell interference, depression, eating disorders, obesity, Chinese Restaurant Syndrome (CRS), birth defects, facial swelling and stroke. Used in Japanese cooking. Leaves a liquorice after taste. On alert in the United States. Approved in the European Union, New Zealand and Australia. **Avoid**

| 960 | Steviol glycosides |
|---|---|
| **Safe** or **Caution** | |

**Colour: Light yellow, odourless powder**
A natural product extracted from the plant: Stevia rebaudiana, Berton. Maybe up to 30 to 320 times sweeter than sucrose. Like all sweeteners, use in moderation. Pure stevia has been used by the South American Indians for centuries and is uncontaminated. Some stevia products on the market contain erythritol or rebaudioside which is extracted using methanol – a highly toxic substance. Check the ingredient label before buying. Is used in many foods where calorie or controlled calorie intake is part of the diet. Used in dietary foods including: breakfast cereal, soups, chocolate and other foods fitting diet programs. Approved in the United States, European Union, New Zealand and Australia. **Safe** or **Caution**

| 961 Caution or Avoid | Neotame |
|---|---|

**Colour: White to off-white powder**
Is between 7,000 to 13,000 times sweeter than sucrose (table sugar). Is sold to bulk food in commercial manufacturing or production. Is used in foods and beverages, chewing gum, carbonated soft drinks, frozen desserts, puddings, fillings, yogurt based foods, baked goods, lollies, sweets and confectionary. Recent studies indicate that neotame is not carcinogenic, mutagenic, teratongenic[244] or associated with any reproductive toxicity. Is however, listed on the food additives list for Romsey Australia.[245] Headaches appear to be the most common complaint. Approved for use in the United States, European Union, New Zealand and Australia. **Caution** or **Avoid**

| 962 Avoid | Aspartame-acesulphame salt |
|---|---|

**Colour: White fine-flowing powder**
Is produced by soaking a mixture of aspartame and acesulfame in an acidic solution. The solution is allowed to dry. Crystals produce the remaining salt. Is highly toxic.[246] Used in chewing gum, pudding mixes, dairy shake mixes, chocolate and pink fizzy drinks. *'Other foods may contain this additive.'*[247] *'It appears that these sweeteners affect the bacteria in the bowel in adverse ways.'*[248] Weizmann

---

[244] A substance or organism that caused malformations in a fetus.
[245] http://romseyaustralia.com
[246] http://www.wotzinurfood.com
[247] http://www.sugar-and-sweetener-guide.com
[248] https://www.weizmann.ac.il

Institute of Science, Rehovot, Israel. (17th September 2014.) See 950 and 951. Also see the recommendation issued by The Centre for Science in the Public Interest, (CSPI). Is linked to cancer. On alert in the United States. Approved in the European Union, New Zealand and Australia. **Avoid**

| 965<br>**Avoid** | **Maltitols**<br>**(i) Maltitol**<br>**(ii) Maltitol syrup or Hydrogenated[249] glucose syrup** |
|---|---|

**Colour: Is a liquid glucose syrup**
Is genetically modified and produced from the starch in plants including wheat, tapioca corn and maize. Is a sugar alcohol, possibly derived from hydrogenated glucose, which is used as a low-calorie sweetener, thickening agent, and texture component used in the production of: chocolates, candies, confectionary, dried fruits, low-joule foods, baked goods, ice cream, chewing gum and coated tablets. During animal (rat) studies there was no foetus toxicity. However, it caused increased tumours in further laboratory animal testing. Is linked to *'bloating, diarrhoea, gas, birth defects, genetic damage.'*[250] Can drastically increase blood sugars. More studies and research is required relating to human consumption of this additive. On alert: all maltitols/maltitol in the United States. On alert: maltitols in the European Union. Approved in New Zealand and Australia. **Avoid**

---

[249] Is to treat with hydrogen through heating and to induce a chemical reaction to a catalyst of nickel, palladium or platinum.
[250] http://thearticlebay.com

| 966 Caution or Avoid | Lactitol |
|---|---|

**Colour: Crystal appearance resembling sugar**

Is a synthetic sugar alcohol and artificial sweetener. Works as an emulsifier when added to manufactured foods. Foods include: ice cream, biscuits, chocolate, chewing gum, sweets (candy), confectionary, cocoa based products, mustards, pickles, jams, jellies, breakfast cereal and baked products. Products having the label: NO ADDED SUGAR, may have this product included. Check the label. Taken in moderation, it supports the bacteria in the colon which supports colon health. Is linked to *'bloating, diarrhoea, gas, birth defects and genetic damage.'* See 965. In some people it may cause stomach cramps and diarrhoea. On alert in the United States. Approved in the European Union, New Zealand and Australia. **Caution** or **Avoid**

| 967 Avoid | Xylitol |
|---|---|

**Colour: White crystalline**

Is a synthetic alcohol sweetener and humectant. In industrial quantities it's derived from wood pulp. Is naturally produced in plums, raspberries, corn and lettuce. Has a low calorie content. Is metabolised in the body while the remainder undergoes fermentation in the large intestine. May cause bloating, Irritable Bowel Syndrome (IBS), kidney stones and gas. Is linked to cancer. May cause diarrhoea and stomach upset. Scientific research has shown tumours in animal testing. Approved in the United States, European Union, New Zealand and Australia. **Avoid**

| 968 **Caution** | Erythritol |
|---|---|

**Colour: White crystalline powder**
Is a naturally modified product found in some fruits and mushrooms. Is a sugar alcohol or (polyol). Is also a stabiliser, bulking agent and sugar substitute. To date, it shows no side effects. The European Union Scientific Committee on Food (SCF), have stated: *'that erythritol is safe for use in foods.*[251] Used in low-joule foods, carbohydrate modified sweets, lollies or candies, chewing gum, ice cream, chocolate and jams. Also used to sweeten dairy desserts, yogurts, hard sweets, candy and confectionary. Large doses may cause nausea. May cause skin rashes, bloating, gas, itching and severe allergic reaction. Like all other additives, professional advice should be sought before adding it to baby and young children's food. On alert in the United States. Approved in the European union, New Zealand and Australia. **Caution**

| 969 **Caution** or **Avoid** | Advantame |
|---|---|

**Colour: Small white tablet**
Is a sweetener that is 20,000 times sweeter than sugar. Developed in Japan made from a chemical composition of aspartame and vanillin – both artificial substances. Used as a general purpose sweetener and flavour enhancer. It's similar to neotame which is based on aspartame. With this, an assumption may be drawn that it can be partially or wholly metabolized by the digestive system. Not yet certified or evaluated. Can be used in high cooking temperatures making it suitable for processed food. May

---

[251] https://www.efsa.europa.eu

have a detrimental effect on gut bacteria and the intestine. Recent studies have revealed, sweeteners can contribute to glucose intolerance.[252] Suitable for people with the genetic disorder: phenylketonuria (PKU). Always check with your health care professional before use. Approved in the United States, European Union, New Zealand and Australia **Caution** or **Avoid**

---

[252] Weizmann Institute of Science

## Your Notes

**Devils: Foaming agents (900 range)**

| Devil Numbers | Additive |
|:---:|:---:|
| **999**<br>Caution or Avoid | (i) Quillaia extract (type 1)<br>(ii) Quillaia extract (type 2) |

**Red to brown liquid or light-brown powder**
Is known as the soap tree. Quillaia is obtained by aqueous extraction from the milled bark of the Quillaia saponaria Molina tree, (Rosaceae family). Products extracted include: glycosides of quillaic acid, polythenols, tannin, sugars and calcium oxalate. Quillaia extract is commercially available. This compound carries lactose, maltitol or maltodextrin. The liquid is usually preserved with sodium benzoate or ethanol.[253] Is used as a foaming agent and emulsifier. Is used in frozen dairy desserts, sweets, candy or confectionary, baked goods, gelatines, puddings and beverages also used as a foaming agent in beer. Is banned in a number of countries. On alert in the United States. Approved in the European Union. On alert in New Zealand and Australia. Caution or Avoid

---

[253] http://files.foodmate.com

**Your Notes**

..............................................................................
..............................................................................
..............................................................................
..............................................................................
..............................................................................
..............................................................................
..............................................................................
..............................................................................
..............................................................................
..............................................................................
..............................................................................
..............................................................................
..............................................................................
..............................................................................
..............................................................................
..............................................................................
..............................................................................
..............................................................................
..............................................................................
..............................................................................
..............................................................................
..............................................................................

## Devils: Additional chemicals and starches (1001 range)

'Acid treated starch is a carbohydrate polymer prepared by treating starch or starch granules with inorganic acids such as sulphuric acid, hydrochloric acid or phosphoric acid, which is later neutralised by the use of sodium hydroxide or sodium carbonate. This causes the starch to partially hydrolyse (breakdown). Starch is a natural polysaccharide derived from roots, the leaves of corn, wheat, potato, rice, tapioca and sago. The properties of acid treated starch change with the heat and acid treatment applied, as does the varying degree of solubility in cold water. **_Acid treated starch is used as a thickener, stabiliser and binder in food_**.'[254]

| Devil Numbers | Additive |
|---|---|
| **1001**<br>**Avoid** | **Choline salts and esters**<br>**(i) Choline acetate**<br>**(ii) Choline carbonate**<br>**(iii) Choline chloride**<br>**(iv) Choline citrate**<br>**(v) Choline tartrate**<br>**(vi) Choline lactate** |
| **Colour: White crystal powder**<br>Cholines are a chief element of biological membranes. Used as an emulsifier. In natural food intake, lecithin is present in many plants and foods including egg yolks and soybean. For mass production, starches can be mechanically extracted and synthesised using hexane[255] extraction. Check for additive type: natural or synthetic and extraction method. Used in multivitamins, sport and energy drinks. Is used in the treatment of Autism as the | |

---

[254] http://mukk.ru

[255] Is a by-product of petroleum and crude oil refinement. Is colourless liquid and hydrocarbon present in petroleum spirit.

product improves brain function and neural circulation. All additives in this number, apart from (iii) choline chloride are on alert in the United States. All additives are on alert in the European Union. All on alert in New Zealand and Australia apart from choline salts and esters. **Avoid**

| 1100 **Caution** | a-Amylase |
|---|---|

**Colour: Brown dense liquid**
Derived from mushrooms or pig pancreas. Is used in bread making and dough products to break down complex sugars such as starch that are found in flour. Is also used as a flavour enhancer in many dough products. Stabilises enzymes and prevents microbial growth. May be toxic to some people. On alert in the United States and the European Union. Approved in New Zealand and Australia. **Caution**

| 1101 **Avoid** | Proteases (i) Proteases (ii) Papain (iii) Bromelain (iv) Ficin |
|---|---|

**Colour: Light tan**
Is an enzyme derived from fig latex but can be derived from a number of sources. Is used as a flour enhancer, flour treatment agent and stabiliser. Used as a flavour enhancer, and meat tenderiser. Also used in alcoholic drinks. Proteases can be teratogenic.[256] Approved in the United States: proteases, (ii) papain, (iii) bromelain. On alert: (i) and (iv). On alert and not approved in the

---

[256] Can disturb the development of the embryo or foetus.

European Union. Approved in New Zealand and Australia. **Avoid**

| 1102 **Caution** or **Avoid** | Glucose oxidase also known as Notatin (GOx) |
|---|---|

**Colour: Off white to brown liquids**
Allows for the catalyses[257] of oxidation to glucose to create hydrogen peroxide. Is used as an additive in dough and bakery products. Also helps to remove oxygen from food packaging or glucose from egg white to inhibit browning. More research required. On alert in the United States and the European Union. Approved in New Zealand and Australia. **Caution** or **Avoid**

| 1104 **Caution** or **Avoid** | Lipases |
|---|---|

**Colour: White to light beige powder**
Are enzymes widely used in the '*…food industry to modify flavour by synthesis of esters of short-chain fatty acids and alcohols which are known flavour and fragrance compounds.' (Macedo et al 2003).*[258] Used in flavour development for: cheese, butter, margarine, milk chocolate and alcoholic beverages. Also used in sweets, candies and confectionary. More research is required to justify the use of this additive in the food industry. On alert in the United States and the European Union. Approved in New Zealand and Australia. **Caution** or **Avoid**

---

[257] Accelerate or cause a reaction by acting as a catalyst.
[258] https://scialert.net

| 1105 **Caution** or **Avoid** | Lysozyme |
|---|---|

**Colour: White odourless powder**
Usually produced from egg white. Can be genetically modified. Is an antibacterial and preservative. Can be responsible for severe allergic reactions. Is used in infant nutrition and pharmaceutical products. Also used as a preservative in hard cheese. Can contribute to severe allergic reactions. More information required. On alert in the United States. Approved in the European Union, New Zealand and Australia. **Caution** or **Avoid**

| 1200 **Caution** | Polydextrose |
|---|---|

**Colour: Light tan solid**
Is a stabiliser, thickening agent and humectant[259] carrier and bulking agent. Is a plasticised mixture of polymer, glucose and sorbitol. May be produced from genetically modified plants. Is used in manufactured baked foods, modified carbohydrates, chocolate, jams, ice cream, low-joule foods and confectionary. May be safe in small doses. Can be a laxative and cause diarrhoea. Not to be given to babies and infants. May be suitable for diabetics. See additive 967. Approved in the United States, European Union, New Zealand and Australia. **Caution**

---

[259] Retains moisture.

| 1201 Avoid | Polyvinylpyrrolidone PVP |
|---|---|

**Colour: Light tan**
Is used as a thickening and stabilising agent. Is made from formaldehyde, acetylene, hydrogen and ammonia which are mainly used in the production of industrial resins, particle board and coatings. Also used in the coatings for tablets and in sweeteners. Is also used in low-joule foods, white wine, some beer, chewing gum and toothpaste. May cause damage to the lungs, kidneys, liver toxicity, allergic reaction and skin irritation. Is also linked to*: 'intestinal blockage, cancer, liver and lung damage. Found in many tablets and capsules which contain vitamins, minerals and herbs. Sold in ordinary shops and health food stores.'*[260] Approved in the United States, European Union, New Zealand and Australia. **Avoid**

| 1400 Caution or Avoid | Dextrin roasted starch |
|---|---|

**Colour: White, yellow or brown powders**
Is a stabiliser and thickener which is gluten-free. Used in commercial bread and bakery products. Dextrin occurs on the surface of bread during baking. It's seen as the golden, crisp crust. This all adds to your desires to eat and want more. Dextrin is also used in batters, food coatings, food glazes, vegetable gum and as a foam stabiliser in beer. Artificial sweetener bases can come from tapioca or corn or possibly from GMO soya. May be used in some digestible baby food, however, the chemicals used in production of the product may not be safe. Check the ingredients. Not fully evaluated for food consumption or safety. Other uses:

---

[260] http://thearticlebay.com

paper coatings, pharmaceuticals, as a pyrotechnic binder, also used in fuel. Approved in the United States. On alert in the European Union. Approved in New Zealand and Australia. **Caution** or **Avoid**

| 1401  **Caution** or **Avoid** | Acid treated starch |
|---|---|

**Colour: White powder**
Is used as a thickening agent. Is gluten-free and added to many foods. Is added to cheese granules as in macaroni cheese or lasagne, gravy granules, commercial pizza; helps in fat replacement in low-fat foods; is added to frozen foods to stop them dripping when defrosted, acts as an emulsifier for French dressing. Forms the shells on many sweets and lollies such as jellybeans and increases the stickiness of batter. *'No known side effects, but not fully evaluated for safety. Foods are made more digestible to babies but the chemicals to create may be harmful.'*[261] On alert in the United States and the European Union. Approved in New Zealand and Australia. **Caution** or **Avoid**

| 1402  **Caution** or **Avoid** | Alkaline treated and modified starch  Also known as Lye or costic soda |
|---|---|

**Colour: White powder**
A product prepared by treating starch granules or starch with sodium or potassium hydroxide. Is used to chemically peel fruit and vegetables. Is used as a thickening agent, is in gluten-free food and added to many other foods. Is

---

[261] http://www.angelfire.com

added to cheese granules as in macaroni cheese or lasagne, gravy granules, commercially produced pizza, helps in fat replacement in low-fat foods. Is added to frozen foods to stop them dripping when defrosted, acts as an emulsifier for French dressing, forms the shells on many sweets and lollies such as jellybeans and increases the stickiness of batter. Also used in chocolate and cocoa processing, caramel colouring and poultry-scalding. Used in soft drink processing and thickening for ice cream. Softening olives: olives are often soaked in a solution of sodium hydroxide. For human consumption and health, more research is required. On alert in the United States and the European Union. Approved in New Zealand and Australia. **Caution** or **Avoid**

| 1403<br>**Avoid** | **Bleached starch** |
|---|---|

**Colour: White powder or granules**
The natural product is modified by enzyme or chemical processing. Is bleached with sulphur dioxide. Used as a thickening agent, emulsifier and stabilising agent in many foods. May be genetically modified. Used in, custards, baby foods, puddings, soups, sauces, salad dressings, wine gums, pie fillings, noodles, pasta and many different sweets, lollies and batter mixes. Not fully evaluated, more testing required. On alert in the United States and the European Union. Approved in New Zealand and Australia. **Avoid**

| 1404 Avoid | Oxidised starch |
|---|---|

**Colour: White fine powder**

Used in foods as a thickening agent, emulsifier and stabiliser. Oxidised starch is broken down by bleaching with sodium hypochlorite or chlorinated bleach. Is used as a vegetable gum; also used in baby foods, jellies, or jelly added sweets, lollies, confectionary, wine gums and batter mixes. Modified starch can be used as a fat substitute in commercial production and the manufacture of yogurts, hard salami, macaroni cheese, lasagne and commercial pizza toppings. The use of chlorine bleach is considered to be unsafe in the use of food production, it can cause caustic burns and is shown to have various levels of carcinogens causing serious cancer conditions. Is linked to: *'high blood cholesterol, pathological changes in the lungs, calcium deposits in the kidneys and stomach. The proven cancer-causing chemicals: epiklorohydrin[262] and propylene oxide[263] have been found in 1404 - 1452.'*[264] On alert in the United States. Not approved in the European Union. Approved in New Zealand and Australia. **Avoid**

| 1410 Avoid | Monostarch phosphate |
|---|---|

**Colour: Dark brown oil**

If made from corn, it may be genetically modified. Used as a thickener, stabiliser and as a vegetable gum which may

---

[262] Is used in the manufacture of plastics, epoxy glues, resins, elestomers and glycerol.

[263] Used in the production of polyurethane plastics.

[264] http://thearticlebay.com

be bleached. Is gluten-free. Used in some baby food, wine gums, jellies, sweets and confectionary. Also used in puddings and batter mixes. No known side effects but is not fully tested or evaluated. However, '*linked to high blood cholesterol, pathological changes in the lungs, calcium deposits in the kidneys, stomach disorders, proven cancer-causing chemicals: epiklorohydrin and propylene oxid.*' Please see 1404. Further testing on this additive is required. On alert in the United States. Approved in the European Union, New Zealand and Australia. **Avoid**

| 1412 **Avoid** | Distarch phosphate |
|---|---|

**Colour: White, off white or canary yellow granular powder**
Used as a thickening agent, stabiliser and emulsifier, also used as a gum. May be bleached. Used in baby foods, jelly-based sweets, lollies and confectionary, wine gums, batter mixes, yogurt, puddings, mayonnaise, canned foods, ice cream, frozen noodles, sauces, salad dressing, seasoning and other commercially manufactured food products. Can be harmful to asthmatics. May also be harmful in baby foods. '*Linked to high blood cholesterol, pathological changes in the lungs, calcium deposits in the kidneys, stomach disorders, proven cancer causing chemical:s epiklorohydrin and propylene oxide have been found in 1404.*'[265] Check the ingredients. Further evaluation and testing needed. On alert in the United States. Approved in the European Union, New Zealand and Australia. **Avoid**

---

[265] http://thearticlebay.com

| 1413 Avoid | Phosphated distarch phosphate |
|---|---|

**Colour: White fine powder**

Is a synthetic additive. Is a food stabiliser, emulsifier, modifier and thickener. Is a resistant starch derived from amylose maize starch. *'Is prepared by treating starch with a phosphorylating agent, trimetaphosphate or phosphor oxychloride and phosphoric acid.'*[266] [267] May be from genetically modified grain products. Is used as a thickener in baby food, wine gums and jelly-based sweets, lollies and confectionary, batter mixes, cola drinks, soft drinks and a wide range of food. See 1400. *'Is linked to high blood cholesterol, pathological changes in the lungs, calcium deposits in the kidneys, stomach disorders. The proven cancer-causing chemicals: epiklorohydrin and propylene oxide have been found in 1404-1452.'*[268] Can be a dangerous additive to asthmatics. Further scientific testing required. On alert in the United States. Approved in the European Union, New Zealand and Australia. **Avoid**

| 1414 Avoid | Acetylated distarch phosphate |
|---|---|

**Colour: White powder with a slight smell of vinegar**

Is a synthetic thickening agent, stabiliser, emulsifier used in the commercial food industry. Also used in pharmaceuticals and in paper production. Can be made from genetically modified grain or vegetable gum, which may be bleached. Is made from potato or maize starch. Is used in soups, sauces, mayonnaise, baby food, jelly-based

---

[266] http://www.wotzinurfood.com
[267] A treatment of phosphates with sulphuric acid.
[268] http://thearticlebay.com

sweets and lollies, wine gums, batter mixes and a wide range of food. As with 1422, it contributes to: 'high blood cholesterol, pathological changes in the lungs, calcium deposits in the kidneys, the proven cancer causing chemicals: epiklorohydrin and propylene oxide have been found in 1404-1452.'[269] Is dangerous for asthmatics. On alert in the United States. Approved in the European Union, New Zealand and Australia. **Avoid**

| 1420 **Avoid** | Starch acetate |
|---|---|

**Colour: White off white or canary yellow**

Used as a thickener, binder, stabiliser and emulsifier. 'Used as a vegetable gum, which may be bleached with phosphoric acid or acetic acid.'[270] Is gluten free. May be produced from genetically modified grain products. Used in some baby foods, wine gums, fillings, batter mixes, egg white mix, some yogurts and dairy-based foods, iced lollies, mixed confectionary, jelly-based lollies and sweets. May be dangerous to asthmatics, causes diarrhoea. 'Is linked to high blood cholesterol, pathological changes in the lungs, calcium deposits in the kidneys, stomach disorders. The proven cancer-causing chemicals: epiklorohydrin and propylene oxide have been found in 1404-1452.'[271] On alert in the United States. Approved in the European Union, New Zealand and Australia. **Avoid**

---

[269] http://thearticlebay.com
[270] http://www.wotzinurfood.com
[271] http://thearticlebay.com

| 1422 Avoid | Acetylated distarch adipate |
|---|---|

**Colour: White, nearly white amorphous powder**
Can be from genetically modified grain. Is a stabiliser, binder, thickener, emulsifier used in many foods, including: baby food, mayonnaise, ketchup, frozen foods, convenience and take away foods, canned foods, dairy products including yogurts, gravies, sauces, dry soup mixes, pâté , fruit preparations, ham brine, salad dressing, seasoning, wine gums, jelly based sweets and lollies, iced lollies, egg white mix and flavoured fruit filling. Also *'adds to high blood cholesterol, pathological changes in the lungs, calcium deposits in the kidneys, the proven cancer-causing chemicals: epiklorohydrin and propylene oxide have been found in 1404-1456.'*[272] Could be dangerous for asthmatics. Babies should not be given food with this additive number. Further testing is required. On alert in the United States. Approved in the European Union, New Zealand and Australia. **Avoid**

| 1440 Avoid | Hydroxypropyl starch |
|---|---|

**Colour: White off white to canary yellow granular powder**
Is a stabiliser, thickener, binder and emulsifier. May be produced from genetically modified grain. Used in yogurt, puddings, mayonnaise, canned foods, ice cream, frozen microwave noodles, sauces, salad dressings and seasoning. *'Linked to high blood cholesterol, pathological changes in the lungs, calcium deposits in the kidneys, stomach disorders, proven cancer causing chemicals:*

---

[272] http://thearticlebay.com

*epiklorohydrin and propylene oxide have been found in 1404-1452.* [273] On alert in the United States. Approved in the European Union, New Zealand and Australia. **Avoid**

| 1442 **Avoid** | Hydroxypropyl distarch phosphate |
|---|---|

**Colour: White off white to canary yellow granular powder**

Is a stabiliser, thickener, binder and emulsifier. Can be produced from genetically modified grain. Used in yogurt, puddings, mayonnaise, canned foods, ice cream, frozen microwave noodles, sauces, salad dressings and seasoning. *'Linked to high blood cholesterol, pathological changes in the lungs, calcium deposits in the kidneys, stomach disorders, proven cancer-causing chemicals: epiklorohydrin and propylene oxide have been found in 1404-1452.* [274] On alert in the United States. Approved in the European Union, New Zealand and Australia. **Avoid**

| 1450 **Avoid** | Starch sodium octenylsuccinate |
|---|---|

**Colour: White to off white to canary yellow granular powder**

Is a thickener, stabiliser, binder and emulsifier. Is a synthetic, may be from genetically modified grain. Used in batter, long-life milk, reduced fat cream, whipping cream and associated products, baby food and infant food, mayonnaise, dairy products, confectionary, sweets, lollies,

[273] http://thearticlebay.com
[274] http://thearticlebay.com

egg white mix, fruit fillings and salad dressings. *Linked to high blood cholesterol, pathological changes in the lungs, calcium deposits in the kidneys, stomach disorders, proven cancer-causing chemicals: epiklorohydrin and propylene oxide have been found in 1400-1456.* See the Article Bay.com. Can cause toxicity, is a probable carcinogen. On alert in the United States. Approved in the European Union, New Zealand and Australia. Avoid

| 1451<br>Avoid | Acetylated oxidised starch |
|---|---|

**Colour: White to off-white powder**

Is a synthetic which is widely used in food-starch applications such as thickening agents, emulsifier and stabilisers. Used in baby food, wine gums, jelly-based sweets, lollies, iced lollies, a range of confectionary, yogurts, egg white mix, commercially manufactured batter, fruit flavoured filling, commercial pizza toppings, cheese granules in macaroni cheese, lasagne and gravy granules. Used in frozen vegetables to stop dripping once defrosted. If extracted from corn, it may be from genetically modified crops. Is an irritant, may be linked to cancer, *'...high blood cholesterol, pathological changes in the lungs, calcium deposits in the kidneys, stomach disorders. Epiklorohydrin and propylene oxide have been found in 1404-1452.'* [275] On alert in the United States. Approved in the European Union, New Zealand and Australia. Avoid

---

[275] http://thearticlebay.com

| 1505<br>Avoid | Triethyl citrate |
|---|---|

**Colour: A colourless, odourless liquid**
Is commercially produced synthetic from citric acid. Used in foods as a flavouring agent. Also used as whipping aid and gum for sports drinks and in egg whites (liquid and dried). Once ingested, has the ability to become an alcohol in the human body. Is also used as a plasticiser for polyvinylchloride and similar plastics. Used in solvents and surface-active agents. Has the ability to interfere with the human brain and nervous system. Contains PFGA, see 620, is a neurotoxin. Approved in the United States, European Union, New Zealand and Australia. **Avoid**

| 1518<br>Avoid | Triacetin |
|---|---|

**Colour: Clear transparent oily liquid**
Manufactured through chemical synthesis and derived from glycerol. Is an emulsifier, humectant, plasticizer and solvent. Also used in the perfume and cosmetics industries. Used as a binder in solid rocket fuels. Is used in the manufacture of tablets and capsules, also used to coat fresh fruit in the United States; also used as an essence in cigarette filters. *'Linked to brain and nervous system disorders and cancer. Is a neurotoxin.'*[276] Approved in the United States, European Union, New Zealand and Australia. **Avoid**

---

[276] http://thearticlebay.com

| 1520 | Propylene glycol or 1,2-propane diol 1,2-dihydroxy propane Methyl ethylene glycol Propane-1,2-diol and brand names |
|---|---|

**Colour: Is a colourless, odourless, clear viscous liquid**

Is a synthetic, petroleum-based, organic compound produced commercially from carbonate and propylene. Is used as a humectant in many foods. As a humectant, lengthens shelf life; is used to coat fruit and vegetables. Used as radiator anti-freeze, wetting agent and dispersing agent. Is used in toothpaste, children's medications and elixirs. Used as an artificial sweetener base in confectionary, chewing gum, a range of different chocolates, food colour essences and in sweetened coconut. Used in hot chilli sauces to enhance their food flavours in global restaurants. *'Has been linked to fatal heart attacks when given intravenously.'*[277] Large doses can be toxic resulting in kidney damage and failure, contributes to depression with reduction and damage of the central nervous system. Has a cancer connection and severe allergic reaction. There has been a total recall of medications containing this additive within the United States. Approved in the United States, the European Union, New Zealand and Australia. **Avoid**

---

[277] https://noshly.com

| 1521<br>Avoid | Polyethylene glycol 8000<br>1,2-propane diol<br>1,2-dihydroxy propane<br>Methyl ethylene glycol<br>Propane-1,2-diol and<br>brand names |
|---|---|

**Colour: Clear white semi-solid or colourless odourless liquid**

Is petroleum-based, commercially produced from propylene[278] and carbonate.[279] *'Can be synthesized from urea and propylene glycol over zinc acetate.'*[280] Is used as a baking agent, flavour enhancer, glazing agent and bread enhancer. Is used in sweeteners and sweetener bases, toothpaste, sweetened coconut, chewing gum, children's medications and elixirs. Also used in chocolate-based confectionary and chocolate. Used in hot chilli sauces in global restaurants to enhance their food flavours. Known to cause renal failure in burns victims. See noshly.com. Linked to fatal heart attacks when given intravenously. Affects the central nervous system, linked to depression and cancer. Is linked to allergies and adverse reactions. Is suspected of being a neurotoxic hazard. A total recall of medications containing this additive within the United States. Approved in the United States, European Union, New Zealand and Australia. **Avoid**

---

[278] Large quantities are used in the production of elastomers, resins and fibres.
[279] Derived from carbon dioxide and carbonic acid.
[280] Synthesis of propylene carbonate from urea used in dietary supplements.

| 1522<br>**Avoid** | Calcium lignosulphonate<br>(40-65) |
|---|---|

**Colour: Light yellow to brown powder**
Using synthetic alcohols obtained from softwood calcium lignosulphonate (40-65). Is used as a carrier for fat soluble vitamins, fruit-based beverages, dairy products, hard sweets, candies and confectionary. Is also used as a water reducing admixture for cement, pesticide suspension, ceramic reinforcing agent, coal water slurry, tanning agents for leather, refractory material binders also used in carbon black granulation. Longitudinal research required. Further reading.[281] Approved in the United States. On alert in the European Union. Approved in New Zealand and Australia. **Avoid**

**Please note: European Union Comments –**

**Codex Committee on Fats and Oils**

'Calcium lignosulphonate liquid should be removed from the Codex list of acceptable previous cargoes. Due to uncertainties, mainly with regard to the composition and toxicity of the low molecular mass fraction, and the fact that the toxicological data are limited to the highly purified 40– 65 calcium lignosulphonate grade and do not cover all grades of calcium lignosulphonate, shipped as previous cargoes, calcium lignosulphonate does not meet the criteria for acceptability as a previous cargo.'[282]

---

[281] http://www.fao.org
[282] https://ec.europa.eu

## Continuing – the poisoning truth – Tom's story

From previously, let's look at some of the food additives found in children's food and drink and add them to the diagram below. By doing this it gives a graphic look at how additives and toxins can build up in a child's system.

## Additives contributing to ADHD and ADD behavioural problems

Listed within this last chapter are over 40 additives that contribute to ADHD, ADD and behavioural problems. For ADHD and ADD, they are:

1)150c, 2) 201, 3)202, 4)203, 5)211, 6)221, 7)223, 8)224, 9)225, 10)251, 11)281, 12)282, 13)283, 14)330, 15)472, 16)620, 17)621, 18)624, 19)625, 20)627, 21) 631.

17)

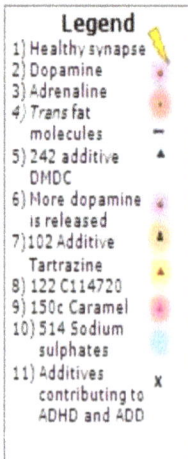

Legend
1) Healthy synapse
2) Dopamine
3) Adrenaline
4) *Trans* fat molecules
5) 242 additive DMDC
6) More dopamine is released
7) 102 Additive Tartrazine
8) 122 C114720
9) 150c Caramel
10) 514 Sodium sulphates
11) Additives contributing to ADHD and ADD

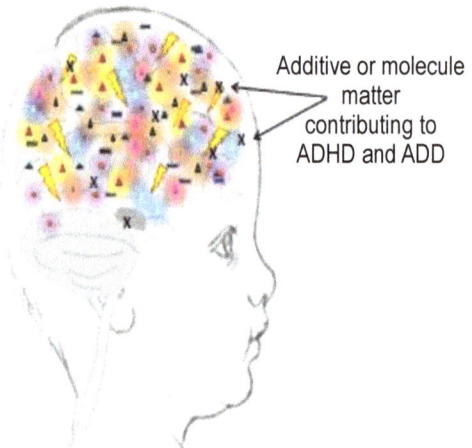

Additive or molecule matter contributing to ADHD and ADD

## Behavioural changes and problems

1)102, 2)124, 3)200, 4)203, 5)211, 6)212, 7)221, 8)223, 9)224, 10)225, 11)249, 12)251, 13)280, 14)281, 15)321, 16)621, 17)622, 18)623, 19)624, 20)627, 21)631, 22)635.

18)

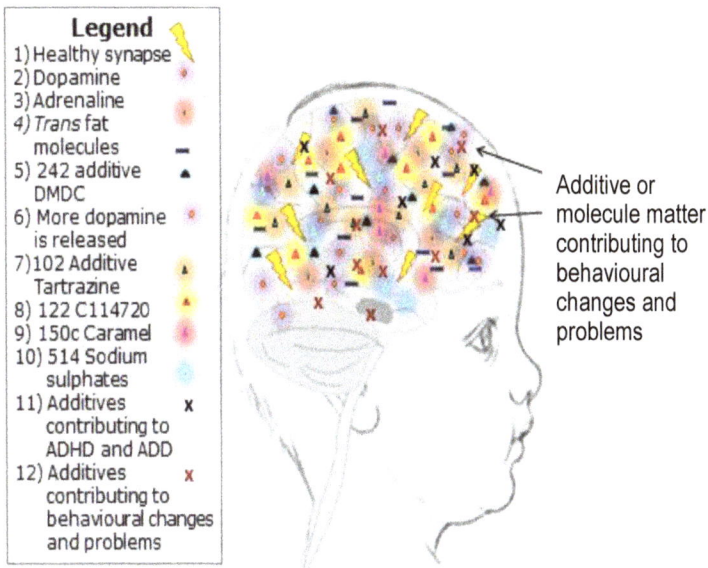

**Legend**
1) Healthy synapse
2) Dopamine
3) Adrenaline
4) *Trans* fat molecules
5) 242 additive DMDC
6) More dopamine is released
7) 102 Additive Tartrazine
8) 122 C114720
9) 150c Caramel
10) 514 Sodium sulphates
11) Additives contributing to ADHD and ADD
12) Additives contributing to behavioural changes and problems

Additive or molecule matter contributing to behavioural changes and problems

An additive or molecule content is so small that we cannot see it with the naked eye, but our body knows it or they are within the human system and reacts accordingly.

Of course food additives don't only impact on the young brain as seen in the above diagram. I have mentioned the young offenders earlier on in the book, these young people were too trying to cope with additives that weren't conducive to their system and their behaviour would highlight the problems they were experiencing. They couldn't say, '*the food I'm eating is poisoning me,*' because they wouldn't have known or been given any of the information I've spoken about in this book.

**For consumers**

> # Check the ingredients label or ask questions of the producer or manufacturer before buying

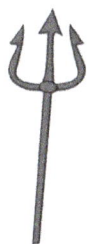

# The Bliss Point

**The Bliss Point of additives**

Without additives being put into manufactured, processed or re-constituted food, the food would become an unsaleable item. Simple, it would have:

- No visual appeal
- No colour appeal
- No texture appeal
- No taste appeal and lastly, it would
- Not be bought a second time.

The processed and food industry only survives because people go and buy the product a second, third, fourth or more times; the product, because of the additive content, has created within the buyer a 'loyalty' factor.

Additive products have been created to work with the 'Bliss Points' of your senses.

**'Bliss Points' with your eyes, taste buds and memory**

- **Eyes –** you see the golden crust of the bread, baguette or bread roll. This has possibly been made using the additive numbers: 102, 170, 200, 213 and other additives
- **The taste buds in your mouth** – remember, your stomach doesn't have taste buds, only your mouth contains these
- And lastly, **your memory**. You remember the mouth-watering experience and want to repeat it time and time again. This is the food industries guarantee to make you buy again and again. **This all relates to the 'pleasure centre' in your brain**.

## Food additives

Food additives are mainly synthetic and created through manipulating the natural growth and building structure of a plant or natural product. They are also made from petroleum, coal tar, a range of polymers and other synthetic substances.

## Most food additives are poison

To create the 'Bliss Point' food manufactures will go to many lengths to enhance either the visual appeal or the taste of their products. Many manufacturers will add coal tar, a by-product of either coal or petrol (both are toxic and carcinogenic). Others use hydrogenation to make their products appealing both visually and through taste.

For example, over thousands of years, bread has been a natural food for civilisations. Now in the Twenty First Century, and with the advancement of technology, bread will have many different ingredients and additives added that are not conducive to the human gut. Simply, once eaten, some additives will accumulate in our bodies because the gut enzymes do not have the ability to break synthetic additives or ingredients down. For food to be adequately broken down gut enzymes have to recognise the molecule; it's a form of communication between the molecule and enzyme that has taken many thousands of years of evolution to develop.

Synthetic or corrupt molecules cannot be disposed of by the human body. These will accumulate in the liver, add to weight gain and obesity showing itself in the thighs, hips and eventually in the brain, heart and other soft organs or areas of the body. This will lead to illness, new diseases and premature deaths.

Additives create **'fake food'**. The food with synthetic or artificial additives has no nutritional value for the body, brain and mind.

# The devil's persuasion

## The devils in food additives

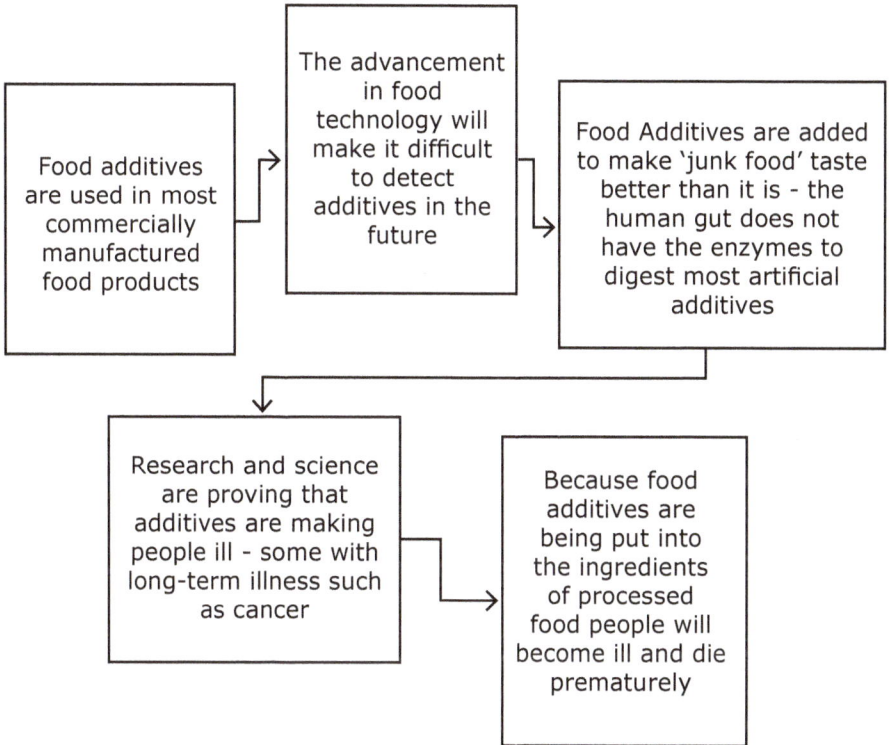

```
┌──────────────────┐     ┌──────────────────┐     ┌──────────────────────┐
│ Food additives   │     │ The advancement  │     │ Food Additives are   │
│ are used in most │ ──→ │ in food          │ ──→ │ added to make 'junk  │
│ commercially     │     │ technology will  │     │ food' taste better   │
│ manufactured     │     │ make it difficult│     │ than it is - the     │
│ food products    │     │ to detect        │     │ human gut does not   │
│                  │     │ additives in the │     │ have the enzymes to  │
│                  │     │ future           │     │ digest most artificial│
│                  │     │                  │     │ additives            │
└──────────────────┘     └──────────────────┘     └──────────────────────┘

        ┌──────────────────────┐     ┌──────────────────┐
        │ Research and science │     │ Because food     │
        │ are proving that     │     │ additives are    │
        │ additives are making │ ──→ │ being put into   │
        │ people ill - some    │     │ the ingredients  │
        │ with long-term       │     │ of processed     │
        │ illness such as      │     │ food people will │
        │ cancer               │     │ become ill and   │
        │                      │     │ die prematurely  │
        └──────────────────────┘     └──────────────────┘
```

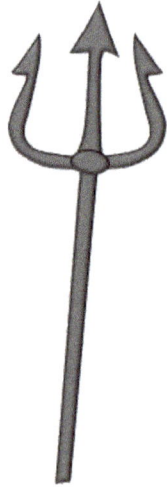

# Devils in
# Our Food

**Your Notes**

..................................................................................

..................................................................................

..................................................................................

..................................................................................

..................................................................................

..................................................................................

..................................................................................

..................................................................................

..................................................................................

..................................................................................

..................................................................................

..................................................................................

..................................................................................

..................................................................................

..................................................................................

..................................................................................

..................................................................................

..................................................................................

..................................................................................

# Chapter ~ Five

*The devil of additives and our DNA – our future generations*

In Chapter One, I briefly spoke of our son becoming a Type One Diabetic. I also mentioned the young offenders and their diet. During her teen years, one of our daughter's was diagnosed with celiac disease. However, the trigger that made me start to write this book, over twelve months ago, was a visit from one of our grandchildren and her constant desire to drink manufactured fruit drinks. In the end, I had to ask myself, '*what is in these things that make a child want to drink this so constantly?*' Her behaviour was prompting me to ask this question. The outcome is now in the previously written pages.

**The devils**

So far, we have seen many devils and not too many angels. That appears to be the way the food manufacturing companies want us to go. However, as consumers, we have the power to make the changes to the food we buy and eat.

This book has not been written about us necessarily but about our children and the future generations that will follow. If we don't do something now, the children of tomorrow will be eating the food conglomerates want them to eat!

This is evident in areas of the world today. Recently seen on television was a documentary of: '**50 Of The World's Best (And Worst) Diets.'**

A mother in the Marshall Islands in the Northern Pacific shared her weekly grocery shopping products with the presenters of the program. Once a seafaring nation, they fished the seas and grew their own crops. For over five decades, the United States conducted over 316 nuclear tests in the region. Now unable to fish or grow the food they need, they rely on imported, frozen, and processed turkey tails for their meat supplies, tinned vegetables and white rice from the United States. The turkey tails are high fat with little to no nutritional value. The tinned food is processed, and the white rice would contain some arsenic.

The mother was aware of the food displayed and the little food benefit it offered her family. She had bought fresh bananas in an attempt to give the family some fresh fruit.

We don't know the outcome of the DNA of the children with such a poor diet, but the program identified the obesity crisis within the community. With such a diet and the little choices in food selection, people will not only become sick but the possibility of their DNA being interfered with, through the food they eat, may only show itself in the future generations!

## DNA

All people and all children need to have their DNA protected. With the case study just given, there seems to be little concern for such an important part of the human system. After the nuclear testing there was an open commercial market to sell 'junk food' to poor people. This is just one case; there would be many thousands of cases similar to this one around the world.

Our DNA has been handed down from our ancestors' and is a birthright. This precious and unique gift needs to be protected for future generations.

Looking carefully from the inside of our systems, our DNA is what makes us unique. From the colour of our eyes, skin colour or hair colour, these are all part of the DNA system.

## So what is DNA?

DNA is an acid which goes by the name deoxyribonucleic. This acid is where our hereditary material, which is within the nucleus, (the centre structure of a cell), exists. The nucleus of the cell is the blueprint. It instructs the cell to live, grow and when to eventually die.

The human body is made up of trillions of cells and each cell carries a percentage of our DNA. Cells vary according to the function they play within the part of the body they serve. Within each cell there lies mitochondria; this, mitochondria provides the energy which allows the cell to do its work.

Cells also need to protect themselves from invading forces. This is done through the work of lysosomes[283] and peroxisomes.[284] Both help in absorbing unrelated bacteria that infest the cell and remove toxic substances harmful to the cell. In order to operate, DNA form pairs. Each pair is known as a 'base pair'. This base pair is attached to a sugar and phosphate

---

[283] A membrane-bound organelle found in many animal cells. An organelle is a specialised sub-unit within a cell.
[284] A microbody sub-unit known as organelle.

molecule. The molecules are given instruction to make protein.

## Our genes

Genes are what makes you, 'you' and me 'me'. Each gene has two copies: one is inherited from our father and one from our mother.

## Tampering with the DNA system

As consumers there is a vast amount of processed food available. We know from research that molecular changes are being made to processed foods. Molecular structure is changed through hydrogenation, petroleum and synthetic additives or through manipulation of genetic modification.

Molecular biology is an interesting field of research. There are many eminent scientists researching how the molecular structure of our bodies work and indeed how the molecular structure of our food works once it's eaten.

Because we cannot see into the future, we have no idea or picture to learn from. We therefore do not know how the health outcomes, behavioural changes for future generations will be affected by the additives, toxins and poisons eaten the 21$^{st}$ Century. However, one thing is evident and science tells us: because of the lack of enzymes within the human gut and system, we cannot discharge some of the additives and their by-products put into manufactured foods.

**In summary**

As adults, we need to act now. It's vital to protect our DNA – we don't want it changed through the manipulation of the food we eat. Our heritage is who we are and our genes keep us aware of this vital component. Science is already making progress into the field of food technology and science. We don't need research done by the food manufactures but by independent research organisations that have an interest in the future and the health of our future generations.

> Becoming food aware is as important as global warming... We need to take action before it's too late...

# The devils of the future

## The value of our DNA

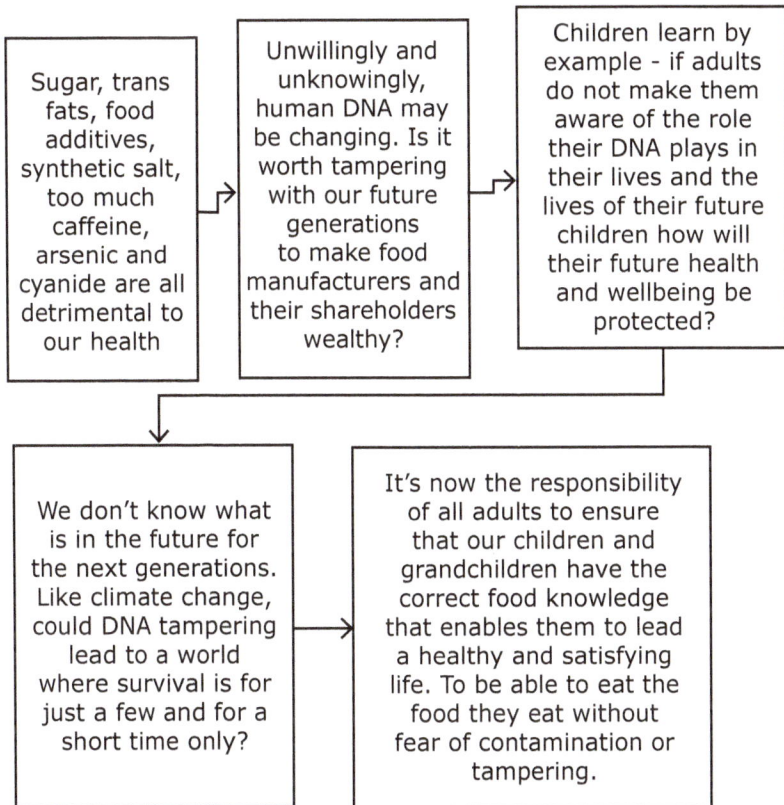

Sugar, trans fats, food additives, synthetic salt, too much caffeine, arsenic and cyanide are all detrimental to our health

Unwillingly and unknowingly, human DNA may be changing. Is it worth tampering with our future generations to make food manufacturers and their shareholders wealthy?

Children learn by example - if adults do not make them aware of the role their DNA plays in their lives and the lives of their future children how will their future health and wellbeing be protected?

We don't know what is in the future for the next generations. Like climate change, could DNA tampering lead to a world where survival is for just a few and for a short time only?

It's now the responsibility of all adults to ensure that our children and grandchildren have the correct food knowledge that enables them to lead a healthy and satisfying life. To be able to eat the food they eat without fear of contamination or tampering.

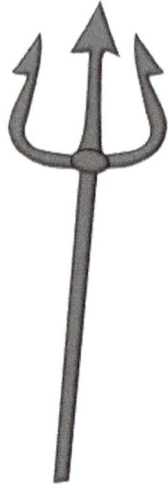

# Devils in
# Our Food

**Your Notes**

..............................................................................
..............................................................................
..............................................................................
..............................................................................
..............................................................................
..............................................................................
..............................................................................
..............................................................................
..............................................................................
..............................................................................
..............................................................................
..............................................................................
..............................................................................
..............................................................................
..............................................................................
..............................................................................
..............................................................................
..............................................................................
..............................................................................
..............................................................................
..............................................................................
..............................................................................

# References

### Dioxin
'Human exposure to dioxins and dioxin-like substances has been associated with a range of toxic effects, including immunotoxicity, developmental and neurodevelopmental effects, and changes in thyroid and steroid hormones and reproductive function. Developmental effects are the most sensitive toxic endpoint making children, particularly breast-fed infants, the population most at risk.' WHO. https://www.who.int/ipcs/assessment/public_health/dioxins/en/

### Dimethyl sulfate
Dimethyl sulfate is an odorless, corrosive, oily liquid with an onion-like odor that emits toxic fumes upon heating. Dimethyl sulfate is used in industry as a methylating agent in the manufacture of many organic chemicals. Inhalation exposure to its vapors is highly irritating to the eyes and lungs and may cause damage to the liver, kidney, heart and central nervous system, while dermal contact causes severe blistering. It is a possible mutagen and is reasonably anticipated to be a human carcinogen based on evidence of carcinogenicity in experimental animals. https://pubchem.ncbi.nlm.nih.gov/

### Esters
'Ester is an organic compound that reacts with water to produce alcohol and acid (organic or inorganic). They are derived from carboxylic acid in which one hydroxyl group is replaced by alkyl group. Common examples for esters includes ethyl ethanoate, ethyl propanoate and methyl butanoate. Its physical properties includes varying boiling points for different esters, solubility

(depends on the chain length), melting point. Polymer form of ester is called polyester which is highly popular in textile industry. Esters are also responsible for aroma of many fruits (apple, banana, pineapple).'
https://www.quora.com/What-is-an-ester-in-chemistry-means

## Glycogen
'Glycogen is a *readily mobilized storage form of glucose.* It is a very large, branched polymer of glucose residues that can be broken down to yield glucose molecules when energy is needed.'
https://www.ncbi.nlm.nih.gov/books/NBK21190/

## Glutamic acid
Is an α-amino acid that is used by almost all living beings and contributes to a biosynthesis of proteins. It is non-essential acid in humans, meaning the body can synthesize it or make its own chemical. Glutamic acid is an excitatory neurotransmitter and is the most found in the vertebrate nervous system.

Please note: PFGA in the 620 - 625 group of additives is synthetic and does not come under the heading of natural glutamic acid.

## Ghrelin
'Ghrelin is a hormone produced in the gut. It is often termed the hunger hormone, and sometimes called lenomorelin. It travels through your bloodstream and to your brain, where it tells your brain to become hungry and seek out food. Ghrelin's main function is to increase appetite. It makes you consume more food, take in more calories and store fat.'
https://www.healthline.com/nutrition/ghrelin#section 1

## Glia

'Glia are non-neuronal cells (i.e. not nerves) of the brain and nervous system. There are a variety of subtypes of glial cells, including astrocytes, oligodendrocytes and microglia, each of which is specialised for a particular function. Glia do not fire action potentials, and because of this were previously thought to be little more than housekeepers that ensured neurons could function properly. This view is now shifting, and astrocytes in particular are recognised as key components of synapses that can influence how we process information.'

https://qbi.uq.edu.au/brain-basics/brain/brain-physiology/what-are-glia

## Hydrogenation

Is to treat with hydrogen. A chemical reaction occurs, usually in the presence of a catalyst such as: platinum, nickel or palladium, between hydrogen ($H_2$) and another compound or element. This method is commonly used to reduce or saturate organic compound/s.

## Ions

'An ion is a charged atom or molecule. It is charged because the number of electrons do not equal the number of protons in the atom or molecule. An atom can acquire a positive charge or a negative charge depending on whether the number of electrons in an atom is greater or less then the number of protons in the atom.'

http://www.qrg.northwestern.edu/projects/vss/docs/Propulsion/1-what-is-an-ion.html

## Lipids

Lipids are molecules that contain hydrocarbons and make up the building blocks of the structure and function of living cells. Examples of lipids include fats, oils, waxes, certain vitamins (such as A, D, E and K), hormones and most of the cell membrane that is not made up of protein. https://www.news-medical.net

## Metalloprotein
Is a generic term for proteins that contain a metal ion. For example: there are 1,000 human proteins in every 20,000 human proteins that contain zinc-binding proteins, although there may be up to 3,000 metallproteins within the area.

## Micarobiome
'The collection of microbes that live in and on the human body is known as the *microbiota*. The *microbiome* refers to the complete set of genes within these microbes. Microbial genes significantly influence how the body operates and even outnumber human genes by a ratio of 100:1. Each of us has a unique microbiota and a unique microbiome. The microbes that live in your body are determined by what you're exposed to and these colonies are constantly in flux. Geography, health status, stress, diet, age, gender, and everything you touch all affect the composition of your microbiota.'
https://www.globalhealingcenter.com/natural-health/what-is-the-microbiome/

## Molecule
'A small mass of matter, (the smallest amount of a substance which can exist alone) an aggregation of atoms specifically a chemical combination of two or more atoms forming a specific chemical substance.'
https://medical-dictionary.thefreedictionary.com/molecule

**Parasympathetic system**

The parasympathetic system is responsible for stimulation of 'rest-and-digest' or 'feed and breed' activities that occur when the body is at rest, especially after eating, including sexual arousal, salivation, lacrimation (tears),urination,
digestion and defecation.

**PFGA**

A new hazardous chemical 620 is also called PFGA or Processed Free Glutamic Acid. This chemical is highly processed and highly refined and 'free' (unbound to other amino acids). PFGA is found in 620-625 additives and contributes to:

- ADD-Attention Deficit Disorder (ADD)
- Attention Deficit Hyperactivity Disorder (ADHD)
- Eating disorders
- Obesity
- Birth defects
- Brain damage
- It destroys brain cells in the area of the hypothalamus
- Chinese Restaurant Syndrome (CRS) with symptoms that are almost identical to a heart attack
- Convulsions
- Depression, including severe depression
- Personality disorders
- Paranoia
- Schizophrenia and
- Suicidal tendencies and other health conditions.

http://thearticlebay.com/en-gb/article/107-food-additives-with-e-numbers

Food awareness can reduce health problems, limit pain and increase life's abundance.

# Further Reading

http://www.angelfire.com

https://www.bbc.co.uk/programmes/articles/1pk5mW
mJXvTQLZYWpN431mW/is-coconut-oil-good-or-bad-
for-your-cholesterol

http://news.bbc.co.uk/2/hi/health/8328377.stm

https://www.choice.com.au

https://www.dangersalimentaires.com

https://www.efsa.europa.eu/en/efsajournal/pub/1650

https://efsa.onlinelibrary.wiley.com/doi/10.2903/j.efs
a.2017.5049

https://efsa.onlinelibrary.wiley.com

http://www.everbum.com

https://www.msn.com/en-au/news/world/teenager-
first-in-uk-to-go-deaf-and-blind-due-to-junk-food-
diet-report-reveals/ar-AAGJlzi?ocid=spartanntp

https://ec.europa.eu/food/sites/food/files/safety/docs
/codex_ccfo_comments_cl-2017-61-fo.pdf
http://www.fao.org/3/y0474s/y0474s11.htm

http://www.foodstandards.gov.au

https://www.foodsweeteners.com

https://www.foodsweeteners.com/microcrystalline-cellulose-side-effects/

http://food-info.net/uk

https://fr-en.openfoodfacts.org/additive/e492-sorbitan-tristearate

https://fr-en.openfoodfacts.org

http://www.fao.org/fileadmin/templates/agns/pdf/jecfa/cta/69/Calcium_Lignosulfonate__40_65.pdf

https://www.getholistichealth.com

https://www.healthline.com

https://healthfully.com

http://www.healthynutritionguide.info/nutrition/food-additives-e-numbers

www.isitbadforyou.com

https://medsafe.govt.nz/profs/Datasheet/s/SodiumBicarbonateinjAFT.pdf

https://members.wto.org/crnattachments/2018/SPS/EEC/18_5639_00_e.pdf

http://mukk.ru
https://nakedwildandfree.com/children-naughty-fruit-shoot/

https://noshly.com/additive/e1520/anticaking-agent-plus/1520/#.XRk_UT8za1t

http://www.nutrientsreview.com

https://www.naturalpedia.com/ammonium-algi-nate-sources-health-risks.html

https://noshly.com

https://www.pressrush.com/author/4882592/jen- krausz

http://www.sugar-and-sweetener-guide.com

https://scialert.net/fulltext/?doi=biotech.2012.100.118

http://www.sci-news.com/medicine/e319-immune-responses-influenza-infection-07071.html

http://thearticlebay.com/en-gb/article/107-food-additives-with-e-numbers

https://truthinlabeling.org

www.truthinlabelling.org

http://www.ukfoodguide.net

http://unitslab.com/node/216

https://www.wisegeek.com

http://www.wotzinurfood.com/e472a-acetic-acid-esters-of-mono-and-diglycerides-of-fatty-acids.html

http://www.wotzinurfood.com/e467-sodium-carboxymethyl-cellulose.html

http://www.wotzinurfood.com/e551-silicon-dioxide.html

https://www.bbc.co.uk/programmes/m000wgcd
Dr Chris van Tulleken

For further information, please see,
Dr Chris van Tulleken's documentary entitled:
BBC One - *What Are We Feeding Our Kids?*

# *Images*

**In appreciation**

Edublogs.org

Image courtesy, minus adaptations,
premiermedicalhv.com

And other mediums

Thank you to Katya Shmaiger and her staff of
Kaligraphic Print Pty Ltd for her support and help.

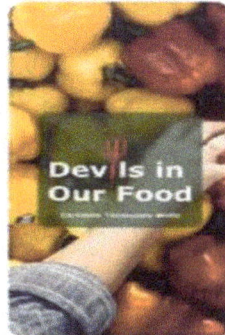

See
Devils In Food
Additives
Your Shopping Handbook

www.how2books.com.au

Shop online

App available: -$1.99

# SEMINARS WORKSHOPS TALKS

## FULL POTENTIAL TRAINING

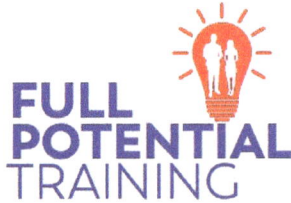

*Full Potential Training is the Working Partner to Books For Reading On Line.Com*

### Devils In Our Food

Hypothesis ~
People can make intelligent decisions about the food they eat once they understand how the manufactured chemistry of the product affects their health.

## Full International Accreditation (CPD)

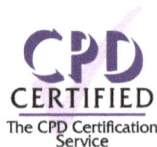

## Lecture

**Performance Criteria and Objective:** is to outline the use and current range of food additives now used in commercially manufactured and processed food.

**Learning Outcome and Application:** how to recognise and understand that many food additives used in the food industry may cause short-term or long-term illness and other health concerns. Suitable for:

- ➢ Food science students and course providers
- ➢ Food educators and supervisors
- ➢ Nutritionists
- ➢ Dieticians
- ➢ Food economists
- ➢ Food manufacturers and producers
- ➢ Restaurants and café owners
- ➢ Government organisations relating to the food industry
- ➢ Universities, Food Schools and Colleges
- ➢ Corporate organisations
- ➢ Other interested groups

Duration: 2.00 hours + 30 minutes for Q & A

## Full International (CPD) Accreditation Workshop

This is a hands-on workshop encouraging discussion points and interaction. There are 5 Modules:

Module 1 – The Devil of Sugar

Module 2 – The Devil of Transfat

Module 3 – The Devils of Table Salt, Caffeine and Rice

Module 4 – The Devils of Food Additives

Module 5 – Our DNA

Performance Criteria and Objective: is to critically investigate the current range of food additives now used in commercially manufactured and processed food.

Learning Outcome and Application: how to recognise and understand that many food additives used in the food industry can be synthetic and are developed to promote taste and appearance and not food goodness. Such additives are proven to cause short-term or long-term illness, other health concerns and negative outcome behaviour.

Duration: 5.00 hours + 1 hour for Q & A

Suitable for:

- ➢ Food science students and course providers
- ➢ Food educators and supervisors
- ➢ Nutritionists
- ➢ Dieticians
- ➢ Food economists
- ➢ Food manufacturers and producers
- ➢ Restaurants and café owners
- ➢ Government organisations relating to the food industry
- ➢ Universities, Food Schools and Colleges
- ➢ Corporate organisations
- ➢ Other interested groups

*For the workshop, delegates are asked to bring a range of packaging that incorporates additive numbers on the ingredient panels.*

**Course materials, handouts and workbook are provided.**

## TALKS

For Schools, Community Groups & Interested Groups

For enquiries and costs, please contact:

admin@fullpotentialtraining.com.au

admin@booksforreadingonline.com